T0227247

Systems Perspective in Beef Practice

Editors

T. ROBIN FALKNER
DALE M. GROTELUESCHEN
JOHN T. GROVES

VETERINARY CLINICS
OF NORTH AMERICA:
FOOD ANIMAL PRACTICE

www.vetfood.theclinics.com

Consulting Editor
ROBERT A. SMITH

July 2022 • Volume 38 • Number 2

ELSEVIER

1600 John F. Kennedy Boulevard • Suite 1800 • Philadelphia, Pennsylvania, 19103-2899

http://www.vetfood.theclinics.com

VETERINARY CLINICS OF NORTH AMERICA: FOOD ANIMAL PRACTICE Volume 38, Number 2
July 2022 ISSN 0749-0720, ISBN-13: 978-0-323-98679-3

Editor: Katerina Heidhausen
Developmental Editor: Axell Ivan Jade M. Purificacion

Veterinary Clinics of North America: Food Animal Practice (ISSN 0749-0720) is published in March, July, and November by Elsevier Inc., 360 Park Avenue South, New York, NY 10010-1710. Subscription prices are $267.00 per year (domestic individuals), $656.00 per year (domestic institutions), $100.00 per year (domestic students/residents), $289.00 per year (Canadian individuals), $686.00 per year (Canadian institutions), $342.00 per year (international individuals), $686.00 per year (international institutions), $100.00 per year (Canadian students), and $165.00 (international students). To receive student/resident rate, orders must be accompanied by name of affiliated institution, date of term, and the signature of program/residency coordinator on institution letterhead. *Clinics* subscription prices. All prices are subject to change without notice. **POSTMASTER:** Send address changes to *Veterinary Clinics of North America: Food Animal Practice*, Elsevier Health Sciences Division, Subscription Customer Service, 3251 Riverport Lane, Maryland Heights, MO 63043. Customer Service (orders, claims, online, change of address): Elsevier Health Sciences Division, Subscription **Customer Service, 3251 Riverport Lane, Maryland Heights, MO 63043. Tel: 1-800-654-2452 (U.S. and Canada); 314-447-8871 (ouside U.S. and Canada). Fax: 314-447-8029. E-mail: journalscustomerservice-usa@elsevier.com (for print support); journalsonlinesupport-usa@elsevier.com (for online support).**

Reprints. For copies of 100 or more, of articles in this publication, please contact the Commercial Reprints Department, Elsevier Inc., 360 Park Avenue South, New York, NY 10010-1710. Tel.: 212-633-3874; Fax: 212-633-3820; E-mail: reprints@elsevier.com.

Veterinary Clinics of North America: Food Animal Practice is covered in *Current Contents/Agriculture, Biology and Environmental Sciences, MEDLINE/PubMed (Index Medicus), and Excerpta Medica.*

Contributors

CONSULTING EDITOR

ROBERT A. SMITH, DVM, MS
Diplomate, American Board of Veterinary Practitioners; Veterinary Research and Consulting Services, LLC, Greeley, Colorado; Veterinary Research and Consulting Services, LLC, Stillwater, Oklahoma

EDITORS

T. ROBIN FALKNER, DVM
Owner, CattleFlow Consulting, Christiana, Tennessee; Beef Cattle Consultant, Elanco Animal Health, Greenfield, Indiana

DALE M. GROTELUESCHEN, DVM, MS
Professor Emeritus, GPVEC-University of Nebraska-Lincoln, Clay Center, Nebraska; Professor Emeritus, University of Nebraska-Lincoln, Lincoln, Nebraska

JOHN T. GROVES, DVM
Owner, Livestock Veterinary Service, Eldon, Missouri

AUTHORS

JADEN M. CARLSON, BS, MS
Graduate Research Assistant, University of Nebraska, School of Veterinary and Biomedical Sciences, Great Plains Veterinary Educational Center, Clay Center, Nebraska

HALDEN CLARK, DVM, MS
Health Stewardship Veterinarian, University of Nebraska-Lincoln, Great Plains Veterinary Educational Center, Clay Center, Nebraska

BRENT CREDILLE, DVM, PhD
Diplomate, American College of Veterinary Internal Medicine; Associate Professor and Director, Food Animal Health and Management Program, Department of Population Health, College of Veterinary Medicine, University of Georgia, Veterinary Medical Center, Athens, Georgia

JOHN DUSTIN LOY, DVM, PhD
Diplomate, American College of Veterinary Microbiology; University of Nebraska-Lincoln, School of Veterinary Medicine and Biomedical Sciences, Nebraska Veterinary Diagnostic Center, Lincoln, Nebraska

T. ROBIN FALKNER, DVM
Owner, CattleFlow Consulting, Christiana, Tennessee; Beef Cattle Consultant, Elanco Animal Health, Greenfield, Indiana

REBECCA A. FUNK, DVM, MS
Assistant Professor of Practice, Great Plains Veterinary Educational Center, University of Nebraska - Lincoln, Clay Center, Nebraska

TIMOTHY J. GOLDSMITH, DVM, MPH
Diplomate, American College of Veterinary Preventive Medicine; Associate Professor, College of Veterinary Medicine, University of Minnesota, St Paul, Minnesota

DALE M. GROTELUESCHEN, DVM, MS
Professor Emeritus, GPVEC-University of Nebraska-Lincoln, Clay Center, Nebraska; Professor Emeritus, University of Nebraska-Lincoln, Lincoln, Nebraska

JOHN T. GROVES, DVM
Owner, Livestock Veterinary Service, Eldon, Missouri

CRAIG A. PAYNE, DVM, MS
University of Missouri, Columbia, Missouri

JASON E. SAWYER, PhD
Associate Professor and Research Scientist, King Ranch Institute for Ranch Management, Texas A&M University, Kingsville, Kingsville, Texas

DAVID R. SMITH, DVM, PhD
Diplomate, American College of Veterinary Preventive Medicine; Diplomate, Epidemiology Specialty; Professor, Department of Pathobiology and Population Medicine, Mississippi State University College of Veterinary Medicine, Mississippi State, Mississippi

GERALD L. STOKKA, DVM, MS
Associate Professor, Extension Veterinarian/Livestock Stewardship Specialist, Department of Animal Science, College of Agriculture, Food Systems and Natural Resources, North Dakota State University, Fargo, North Dakota

BENJAMIN L. TURNER, PhD
Associate Professor, Department of Agriculture, Agribusiness, and Environmental Science, King Ranch Institute for Ranch Management, Texas A&M University-Kingsville, Kingsville, Texas

BRIAN VANDER LEY, DVM, PhD
Diplomate, American College of Veterinary Preventive Medicine; Associate Professor, Veterinary Epidemiologist, University of Nebraska-Lincoln, School of Veterinary Medicine and Biomedical Sciences, Great Plains Veterinary Educational Center, Clay Center, Nebraska

ROBERT W. WILLS, DVM, PhD
Diplomate, American College of Veterinary Preventive Medicine; Diplomate, Epidemiology Specialty; Professor, Department of Comparative Biomedical Sciences, Mississippi State University College of Veterinary Medicine, Mississippi State, Mississippi

KIMBERLY A. WOODRUFF, DVM, MS
Diplomate, American College of Veterinary Preventive Medicine; Diplomate, Epidemiology Specialty; Associate Clinical Professor, Department of Clinical Sciences, Mississippi State University College of Veterinary Medicine, Mississippi State, Mississippi

AMELIA R. WOOLUMS, DVM, MVSc, PhD
Diplomate, American College of Veterinary Internal Medicine, Diplomate, American College of Veterinary Microbiology; Department of Pathobiology and Population Medicine, Mississippi State University, Starkville, Mississippi

Contents

A system is a set of interconnected elements that are organized in such a way to achieve a purpose. Structure and feedback are fundamental properties of all systems and determine system behavior—whether successful or failed. Systems thinking is a methodology used to create structural explanations for why things are happening so we are in a better position to identify long-term strategies that will fundamentally improve system performance. This article addresses the origins of systems thinking and briefly describes a methodology that has been used primarily in business management but has application in veterinary medicine as well.

Managing beef cattle health across a segmented production and marketing system can be thought of as a perplexing problem due to the counterintuitive responses of the system to existing management strategies. The process of thinking in systems to recognize and develop systems thinking archetypes is emphasized. The 2 cases discussed are brought together to explore deeper but often unrecognized structure that contributes to reinforcing problematic behavior, the structure of mental models. Training in systems thinking and system dynamics modeling equips the scientist to translate within and between scientific disciplines, a much-needed skill for addressing current and emerging beef production problems.

The management and care of livestock can be integrated with a stewardship philosophy and a systems approach to health and wellness. Stewardship is the responsible management of things entrusted to one's care. This philosophic approach means that every resource in livestock production, the land, livestock, and people, must be considered in the care and feeding of livestock and the practice of veterinary medicine. The systems thinking discipline is a set of synergistic investigative skills, used to improve the capability of identifying and understanding complex adaptive systems, predicting their behaviors, and devising modifications to them to produce desired changes.

knowledge of simple linear relationships. Beef production systems are complex adaptive systems and decisions and policies throughout the system can positively or negatively affect the health of cattle. Those decisions may occur far removed in time or place from the health event and may be logical in the context of other factors in the system. Causal loop diagrams and stock and flow models are tools for sharing and testing thoughts about the ways systems might behave.

Beef production intensification efforts have included pursuing highly productive genetic lines, increasing herd size, and timing calving season to target marketing opportunities. Changes like these may have incentivized concentration of animals during calving and led to accumulation of risk factors for neonatal calf diarrhea. The Sandhills Calving System (SCS) is an example of a system modification at a point of leverage that has been shown to prevent neonatal calf diarrhea. The development of the SCS can serve as an example of several Systems Thinking concepts.

Despite evidence-based "improvements" in animal health products and management, losses to bovine respiratory disease have increased with associated animal wastage, welfare concerns, and antimicrobial use; questioning the fitness of current disease-centric paradigms for improving critical outcomes in complex adaptive systems. Systems thinking is used to model a paradigm shift from mental models based on management of failure outcomes in a flawed pass/fail dichotomy to one of managing success outcomes on a continuum. In the proposed wellness paradigm, the notion of health as absence of disease is rejected and replaced with perspective of disease as symptomatic of systems insufficiently supporting wellness.

This chapter provides an introductory look into the practical application of the principals of systems thinking as a methodology to gain deeper understanding of the nature of bovine respiratory disease (BRD) in current North American beef production models. The "limits to success" archetype is used to explore the dynamic relationship between technological BRD mitigation improvements and the resultant adaptive changes made by the system. The chapter concludes, by using the tragedy of the common archetype, with an investigation into how the common shared resource of antimicrobials can be damaged and depleted over time.

Beef cattle veterinarians provide services to the increasingly complex beef industry system. Systems thinking offers pathways to better understand and communicate ranges of issues such as prevailing mental models, importance of match quality relative to clientele needs, and identification of leverage to better adapt and continually improve. Thinking in systems identifies and helps us to understand patterns or structures that are organized and interconnected that result in the outcomes observed and experienced in the practice of beef cattle veterinary medicine.

VETERINARY CLINICS OF NORTH AMERICA: FOOD ANIMAL PRACTICE

SERIES OF RELATED INTEREST

Veterinary Clinics: Equine Practice
https://www.vetequine.theclinics.com/

THE CLINICS ARE NOW AVAILABLE ONLINE!
Access your subscription at:
www.theclinics.com

Preface

Perspectives on the Practical Applications of Systems Thinking and System Dynamics Theory in Beef Practice

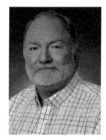
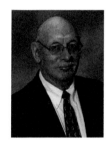
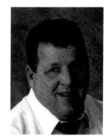

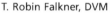

T. Robin Falkner, DVM   Dale M. Grotelueschen, DVM, MS   John T. Groves, DVM

Editors

Undeniably, an unabating challenge confronting the veterinary profession as a whole and, in the case of this issue, beef practitioners, is the ability and willingness to continually adapt fundamental paradigms regarding the nature of "practice" in ways that reinforce high levels of professional relevance, not just to the beef cattle industry but also to the complex adaptive system to which it is inexorably interconnected. More directly stated: Veterinarians involved with beef cattle production are tasked with coevolving in conjunction with a larger system to meet the challenges of "fitness" over time.

The broad and diverse knowledge required for successful rural and agriculturally based practice by previous generations of veterinarians has most surely played a key role in the resilience of the profession over time. The broad knowledge of the general practitioner grew in depth based on the needs of the system. Veterinarians trained in individual animal medicine advanced over time by developing population-based practice models that focus on herd health and production medicine. It is difficult to overemphasize the impact of these advancements on the veterinary profession; however, in our rapidly changing and increasingly complex world, it would be myopic not to embrace the necessity of continuous improvement, not only in our knowledge but also to our approaches to complex challenges facing the profession and our clients. This includes "old challenges" that have resisted our "old approaches," and "new challenges" that emerge, both those that were there but unseen by our "old eyes" and new ones that appear, often as a consequence of past solutions we applied without a sound systems perspective on the potential sequalae of our efforts.

Vet Clin Food Anim 38 (2022) xi–xiii
https://doi.org/10.1016/j.cvfa.2022.03.004
0749-0720/22/© 2022 Published by Elsevier Inc.

vetfood.theclinics.com

With deference to Donella Meadows,[1] scientist and pioneering systems educator, whose book, *Thinking in Systems: A Primer*, is a foundational introduction to systems concepts, we propose for your consideration the concept of "Practicing in Systems" as an opportunity for the continued advancement of veterinary practice. We propose that the addition of proficient SystemsThinking veterinarians to the professional community will enhance our ability to maintain "fitness" and "relevance." For some, the concepts and examples shared in this book will resonate powerfully and naturally; for others, the Systems Thinking and Dynamics disciplines may be perceived as somewhat abstract and impractical. Regardless of the group in which the reader finds themself, it is our contention that increased literacy in systems concepts has high utility for our profession. In addition, for a subset of veterinarians, pursuit of additional training in and application of the systems disciplines can enable significant evolutionary progress for veterinary medicine.

The disciplines of System Thinking and System Dynamics have been addressed, although sparingly, in the veterinary literature. Forward-thinking writers have introduced the concepts and their potential for application in the practice of our profession as well as applications in systems to which we are interconnected. Not long after the turn of the millennia, informal discussions among veterinary colleagues familiar with systems concepts became more frequent. Central to many of those discussions were issues related to resources for learning and training. During recent years, a number of seminars and continuing education offerings at regional and national veterinary meetings, as well as publications, have continued growth and interconnections. These have been helpful in assembling a group of contributors we consider foremost in the integration of systems concepts into our profession.

Veterinary-specific resources for those interested in further advancement in Systems Thinking and practice are for all practical purposes nonexistent, and our effort here is modest and incomplete. However, we hope it serves as a stimulus for additional work. For those so inclined to invest in self-education, there are resources available in the references of the articles of this issue.

We sincerely hope this issue of *Veterinary Clinics of North America: Food Animal Practice* will stimulate readers to learn further and begin to implement, thereby discovering how this discipline might increase "fitness" and "relevance" necessary for adaptation and advancement in veterinary practice and the beef industry.

T. Robin Falkner, DVM
Cattleflow Consulting and
Elanco Animal Health
2404 Walnut Grove Road
Christiana, TN 37037, USA

Dale M. Grotelueschen, DVM, MS
University of Nebraska–Lincoln
School of Veterinary Medicine and
Biomedical Sciences
PO Box 156
Harvard, NE 68944, USA

John T. Groves, DVM
Livestock Veterinary Service
P.O. Box 353
917 South Aurora Street
Eldon, MO 65026, USA

E-mail addresses:
rfalkner@bellsouth.net (T.R. Falkner)
dgrotelueschen@unl.edu (D.M. Grotelueschen)
john@livestockvetservice.com (J.T. Groves)

REFERENCES

1. Meadows Donella, D. Wright, ed. Thinking in systems: a primer. London: Earthscan; 2009.

Fundamentals of Systems Thinking

Craig A. Payne, DVM, MS

KEYWORDS

• Feedback • Structure • Systems thinking • Veterinary

KEY POINTS

- A system is a set of interconnected elements that are organized in such a way to achieve a purpose.
- Structure and feedback are fundamental properties of all systems and determine system behavior.
- Systems thinking is a methodology that is used to create structural explanations for system behavior.

INTRODUCTION

The veterinary profession is immersed in complex systems. Economic, regulatory, business, cultural, environmental, and biological systems are all intertwined, which creates levels of complexity that are difficult to comprehend and generates results that, at times, seem to defy sensible explanation.

Systems thinking is a term commonly used to describe a methodology for analyzing complex systems. However, there is no universally accepted method so it may have different meanings to different people.

The purpose of this article is to introduce a form of systems thinking that has been used worldwide in business management and other disciplines. It will begin with the origins of this particular form of systems thinking; then a definition of systems thinking will be provided; and it will conclude with a brief description of the methodology. Some of the concepts presented in this article will also be encountered elsewhere in this edition and are used in other forms of systems thinking as well.

ORIGINS OF SYSTEMS CONCEPTS

Reductionism is the philosophy that deconstructing a system into its basic elements and studying the properties of those elements is the best way to understand it. This has been the primary approach to scientific discovery for centuries[1] and dates back to at least the 17th century, when Descartes discussed the idea in his *Discourse on Methods*.[2]

University of Missouri, S132 ASRC, 920 East Campus Drive, Columbia, MO 65211-5300, USA
E-mail address: payneca@missouri.edu

Vet Clin Food Anim 38 (2022) 165–178
https://doi.org/10.1016/j.cvfa.2022.02.001
0749-0720/22/© 2022 Elsevier Inc. All rights reserved.

vetfood.theclinics.com

There is no general consensus regarding the origins of systems concepts. However, Ludwig Von Bertalanffy, an evolutionary biologist, has been recognized as one of the pioneers in the modern systems movement.[3] He concluded that growth and change of living organisms could be best explained by the interaction of their parts and that the traditional linear, cause and effect explanations previously offered were insufficient.[4] He proposed "the system theory of the organism" in *Kritische Theorie der Formbildung* (English translation: *Modern Theories of Development*), which laid the foundation for what would later be known as the general systems theory.[5]

Interest and research in systems flourished after World War 2. Individuals from the fields of general systems theory, cybernetics, complexity theory, systems dynamics and others helped shape the ideas surrounding systems.[6] Although no one individual can take credit for systems concepts, there were a few who played a significant role in creating awareness and adoption of the concepts beyond their particular field. One such individual was Jay Forrester.

ORIGINS OF SYSTEMS DYNAMICS

This section is *adapted from* Forrester, JW. The beginning of system dynamics. In: Banquet talk at the international Systems Dynamics Society. 1989. Available at: https://web.mit.edu/sysdyn/sd-intro/D-4165-1.pdf. Accessed September 7, 2021; with permission.

Jay Forrester grew up on a cattle ranch near Anselmo, Nebraska. After high school, he enrolled in the engineering college at the University of Nebraska, completing his degree in 1939. From there he accepted a research assistantship in the Servomechanisms Laboratory at the Massachusetts Institute of Technology (MIT), where he developed feedback control mechanisms for military equipment. In time, he progressed from research assistant to faculty member to director of the MIT Digital Computer Laboratory.

The year 1956 was a turning point in Forrester's career. The MIT Sloan School of Management, which had started four years earlier, offered him the opportunity to apply his engineering knowledge to business management. He was given a year to determine where he should focus his efforts and decided the greatest impact would be researching why some businesses succeed and others fail.

Shortly thereafter, Forrester had a chance encounter with executives from General Electric. They were looking for answers as to why a household appliance plant in Kentucky would at times be running three or four shifts and a few years later need to lay off half of the employees. Typical business cycles were often implicated that did not seem to explain the entirety of the problem.

Using pencil, paper, and the information he collected, Forrester created a model of the inventory control systems. From this, it was determined that the underlying cause was not external factors but that the internal structure and decision-making policies at the plant created an unstable system. This marked the beginning of the field of system dynamics, which uses computer simulation modeling based on feedback systems theory for the purposes of determining strategy and designing policies.[7] Forrester would go on to use system dynamics to explore complex issues outside of business management resulting in publications such as *Urban Dynamics* in 1969 and *World Dynamics* in 1971.

SYSTEM DYNAMICS TO SYSTEMS THINKING

Extensive work in system dynamics in the 1960s, which continues to this day, has led to a form of systems thinking that has become recognized worldwide in business management and beyond. The concepts were initially developed for use when creating system dynamic models and a way to communicate insights gained from those models. In time, the concepts evolved and are now used to reach a wider audience who are less likely to engage in the simulation modeling methods associated with system dynamics. Many individuals and organizations were involved in this effort, all of whom were connected to Jay Forrester. The following are considered some key contributors:

- Dana (Donella) Meadows: Was a research fellow at MIT from 1969 to 1972 and served as lecturer at Dartmouth College from 1972 until her untimely death in 2001. Her books, *Limits to Growth* and *Thinking in Systems* along with a weekly column, brought key ideas of systems thinking to the larger public.
- Peter Senge: Received MS and PhD from MIT and cofounder of Innovation Associates and lecturer at MIT. Author of *The Fifth Discipline: The Art and Practice of a Learning Organization* and coauthor of *The Fifth Discipline Fieldbook*. These books popularized the concepts of systems thinking in business management.
- Consulting/training firms Gould Kruezer Associates and Innovation Associates have been instrumental in the evolution of the tools and practices of systems thinking.
- Pegasus Communications, founded by Daniel Kim and Colleen Lannon, has published many different materials on the practice and application of systems thinking, and organized an annual conference where ideas could be shared. The Omidyar Group purchased the assets in 2013 and the publications are now found at https://thesystemsthinker.com, which is considered to be where the main body of published work on systems thinking resides.

DEFINITION OF SYSTEMS THINKING

Donella Meadows, author of *Thinking in Systems*, described a system as "an interconnected set of elements that is coherently organized in a way that achieves something."[8] Structure and feedback are fundamental properties of all systems. Structure is not an organizational chart, workflow, or process as some may think but is the interrelationships that exist among the elements.[9] The elements may be environmental, biological, economic, policies, cultural norms, individual mental models, and so on, and they are inextricably linked. As a result, a change in one element affects other elements in the system, and their response creates feedback that influences the first element. This cycle repeats again and again thereby determining overall system behavior, whether it is growth, stability, decay, success, or failure.[10]

(Sidebar) "Systems are perfectly designed to achieve what they are achieving right now". Peter Stroh, *Systems Thinking for Social Change.*[11]

Systems thinking is the methods and tools we use to create structural explanations for why things are happening so we can identify strategies to improve system performance.[12] It helps us think differently about complex systems and reveals the unintended consequences of actions, policies, and behaviors.[12] **Table 1** demonstrates how we tend to think about problems versus the systems thinking perspective.

Finally, systems thinking is the most effective when applied to chronic problems that resist change.[11] It seldom provides a single answer to a problem but instead reveals the possible choices we have to fundamentally improve system performance.[13]

SYSTEMS THINKING METHODOLOGY

As mentioned previously, systems thinking helps us create structural explanations for what we observe. The iceberg is used to represent the steps that get us to that point

(**Fig. 1**). This analogy is appropriate because systems, like icebergs, have a portion that is easy to see, which includes events, trends, and patterns. However, these are merely symptoms and the underlying structure creating the symptoms is much more difficult to appreciate. As we move down the iceberg with the use of systems thinking, we develop a deeper understanding of the issue.

The iceberg also serves as a reminder why it is important to focus our attention on structure. Individuals who see the world as only a series of events tend to be reactionary; fixing problems as they arise but not addressing the underlying cause so the problem re-emerges later. Focusing on trends and patterns offers more insight because we can anticipate or forecast what may happen and plan accordingly. However, systems evolve and adapt, and conditions change, so historical trends may not be predictive of future outcomes. By focusing on structure, we develop an understanding of the true nature of the problem and are in a position to create fundamental change.

Systems thinking is the most effective when done as a group exercise and key stakeholders impacted by the issue are invited to participate. The process begins with describing events or what has occurred. This is an opportunity for everyone to share their perspective on what happened, some of the key crises or events, why it is a problem, and what the results have been when changes have been attempted in the past.[12]

The next step is describing trends and patterns or what has been occurring. Ideally, there are three to five key variables selected from the events and a graph is generated showing past trends and possibly where it is headed if change does not occur.[12] Graph lines may be quantitative or qualitative and precision is not necessarily as important as the trend itself—whether increasing, decreasing, or oscillating. This provides the first insight into system behavior.

At this point, it might be beneficial to create a shared vision of what it looks like once the issue is resolved. This increases awareness of the current reality[14] and will be

Table 1
How we tend to think versus systems thinking perspective

How We Tend to Think	Systems Thinking Perspective
The connection between problems and their causes is obvious and easy to trace.	The relationship between problems and their causes is indirect and not obvious.
Others (either within or outside the organization) are to blame for our problems and must be the ones to change	We unwittingly create our own problems and have significant control or influence in solving them by changing our behavior.
A policy designed to achieve short-term success will also assure long-term success.	Most quick fixes either make no long-term difference or actually make matters worse in the long-term.
To optimize the whole, we must optimize the parts.	To optimize the whole, we must improve the relationship among the parts.
The best way to implement change is aggressively tackle many independent initiatives simultaneously.	Target and orchestrate a few key changes over time.

From Goodman M. Introduction to systems thinking. In: John B. Armstrong lectureship in systems thinking proceedings. Innovation Associates Organizational Learning. 2011;2(11):1.6; with permission.

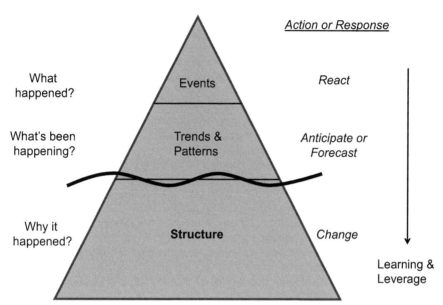

Fig. 1. Systems thinking framework: the iceberg analogy. (*Adapted from* Goodman M. Systems thinking framework. In: John B. Armstrong lectureship in systems thinking proceedings. Innovation Associates Organizational Learning. 2011;2(11):2.8; with permission.)

important when identifying structure—when we know what we want, it's easier to describe what we have.[13]

This is also a good time to develop a focusing question which will be answered in step three. This provides an actionable item and helps you determine the part of system structure you should focus on initially.[11] Keep in mind that it is not uncommon for this question to change as you develop a deeper understanding of the issue.

The third step is identifying structure. Here you describe why this problem happens, what are the forces or pressures at work, what is perpetuating or exacerbating the problems, and mental models involved.[12] Unique to this step is the use of causal loop diagrams or archetypes to describe the structure.

Causal Loops

Many of us are conditioned to analyze and solve problems in a linear, step-by-step fashion[15]; A affects B, which affects C and so on. What we may be less accustomed to is thinking about feedback—how B may affect A and how C may affect B or A. Again, structure is not only the interconnections between elements but how feedback influences the elements. Causal loops are used to convey this and makes thinking visible. From any element, you can draw a line to another element demonstrating feedback and reveal cycles that repeat themselves time and time again making a situation better or worse.[16]

There are two types of causal loops—reinforcing and balancing. With reinforcing loops, the behavior we see is amplification.[11] When an element in the cycle increases/decreases it creates a chain reaction through the other elements and the feedback from the chain reaction causes even more of an increase/decrease in the first element.[12] This cycle repeats over and over again creating either a virtuous or vicious cycle. The story of the virtuous cycle is growth whereas that of the vicious cycle is collapse (**Fig. 2**).

Fig. 3 is an example of a reinforcing loop that may be virtuous or vicious. If a company invests profits in research and development, it increases innovative products or services in the marketplace. This leads to increased sales; profits increase, and more investment can be made in research and development. This cycle repeats thereby growing the business. Change the influence to decrease and the company struggles to survive.

Regarding balancing loops, the behavior observed is that of oscillation (**Fig. 4**). As an element within the chain increases, another element responds with an opposite force to maintain equilibrium at a desired point or condition. The story of the balancing loop is that of constraints, limits, and self-regulation.[12]

Fig. 5 is an example of a balancing loop that many of us are familiar with. As cattle prices trend higher, national herd size increases. Beef supplies also increase but this puts a downward pressure on cattle prices and the national herd size begins to contract.

To improve communication, loops often contain notations. R is used to indicate a reinforcing loop and B for a balancing loop. The direction of influence can also be placed next to an arrow connecting two elements. A plus sign or S is used to represent that the influence is in the same direction and a minus sign or O to indicate that the influence is in the opposite direction. A rule of thumb is that a balancing loop will contain an uneven number of minuses or Os.[17]

A final notation to include are time delays. This is often represented by two parallel lines across the arrow where a delay exists and it is only necessary to include delays that are significant relative to other delays in the loop.[13] For example, a significant delay in the cattle price cycle would be between cattle prices and national herd size.

Recognizing delays is critical because of their significant influence on systems. They make it much more difficult to link cause and effect as the consequences of an action or behavior may take weeks, months, or years to emerge. This prevents positive reinforcing behaviors from ever gaining momentum, allows negative reinforcing behaviors to grow unchecked, or generates wide oscillations when a system overshoots its target only to overcompensate in the opposite direction sometime later.[12]

Exponential growth, which is a characteristic of reinforcing loops,[17] further blurs the connection between cause and effect. Problems go undetected for extended periods of time only to be recognized once they are spinning out of control. Blame is often assigned to recent events because of exponential growth bias, which is the tendency for humans to underestimate the compounding of exponential growth.[18]

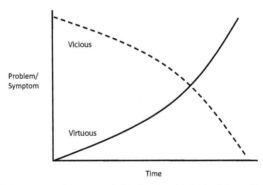

Fig. 2. Vicious and virtuous cycle pattern of behavior. (*Adapted from* Goodman M. Systems language. In: John B. Armstrong lectureship in systems thinking proceedings. Innovation Associates Organizational Learning. 2011;2(11):3.4; with permission.)

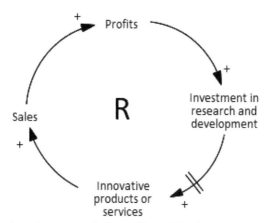

Fig. 3. Reinforcing loop: investment in Research and Development.

Archetypes

The causal loops presented so far are the basic building blocks of structure. Models that sufficiently explain structure are often a combination of interconnected reinforcing and balancing loops.[11] Such models are created with model simulation software; however, many do not have the skills necessary to engage in that process. An alternative is to use archetypes to visualize the underlying structure.

Archetypes are generic patterns of behavior that have been identified to occur frequently within systems.[19] They are a specific combination of reinforcing and balancing loops that help facilitate recognition, understanding and diagramming of system structure.[13]

There is debate on how many archetypes exist, but the ones discussed most often are Fixes that Backfire, Shifting the Burden, Limits to Success, Escalation, Drifting Goals, Success to the Successful, Tragedy of the Commons, and Accidental Adversaries. It is beyond the scope of this article to present each archetype, but two examples are provided to introduce the concept.

Fixes that Backfire is a story of unintended consequences[11] in which a quick fix is applied that works in the short term, but the fix has an unforeseen consequence making the symptom worse in the long term.[12] Unfortunately, we fail to recognize the connection between the fix and the consequence so we apply it again and again

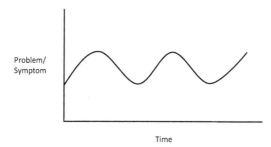

Fig. 4. Balancing loop pattern of behavior. (*Adapted from* Goodman M. Systems language. In: John B. Armstrong lectureship in systems thinking proceedings. Innovation Associates Organizational Learning. 2011;2(11):3.14; with permission.)

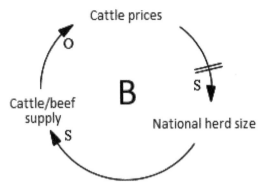

Fig. 5. Balancing loop: cattle price cycle.

without making fundamental improvements.[20] The configuration of this archetype is a balancing loop, which represents the fix, embedded in a reinforcing loop, which represents the unforeseen consequence.

Fig. 6 is an example. Focusing on the top balancing loop first—a business that is experiencing financial difficulty responds by reducing inputs to improve the profitability. This appears to work temporarily, but poor profitability continues to be an issue and is apparently getting worse.

The reason for this is explained by the reinforcing loop. Reducing inputs has the unintended consequence of negatively affecting production, which in turn negatively affects profitability. The fix is applied again because the business does not recognize the impact of reducing inputs due to the significant time delay and profitability is further affected. The pattern of behavior seen over time would be similar to what is found in **Fig. 7**.

The second archetype, Shifting the Burden, is a situation in which a long-term solution has been identified but it is difficult to implement so a quick fix is applied to address the problem.[19] What is not apparent is that the fix has a side effect that

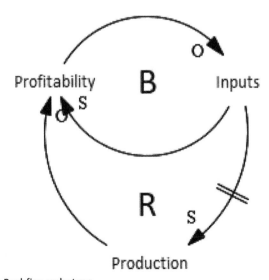

Fig. 6. Fixes that Backfire archetype.

undermines the effectiveness of the long-term solution leading to a dependency on the fix.[12] This is also known as the story of addiction. The basic configuration of this archetype is two balancing loops, with the top loop being the quick fix, the bottom loop being the long-term solution, and an outside reinforcing loop which represents the side effect of the quick fix.

Fig. 8 is an example. In this scenario, a company seems to always be behind with meeting customer demands because of high employee turnover. Employees complain that they have not been adequately trained in their position, become frustrated, and leave within a year or two. Training policies have been implemented, but work continues to pile up and turnover continues to be a problem.

The bottom balancing loop shows why training should be an effective long-term strategy. As customer demand increases, employees are equipped to handle the challenges thereby improving job satisfaction/retention and customer demands are met. However, the top balancing and outside reinforcing loop show why this strategy hasn't been effective. Supervisors feel it is necessary to intervene when customer demand is high to keep the business running. This does temporarily address the issue of customer demand, but the unintended consequence is they devote little time to training so employees are not prepared to deal with high demand and job satisfaction erodes overtime. With each pass, the company gets further behind, but the quick fix is applied again and again because it has been effective, even though temporarily. The pattern of behavior may be similar to what is seen in **Fig. 9**.

Before moving on to the final aspect of identifying structure, some additional comments about archetypes are warranted. Archetype templates provide a good starting point for identifying structure, especially for those new to systems thinking. However, they often require additional loops to sufficiently describe structure. In addition, several archetypes may be identified and a decision will eventually need to be made regarding which one offers the best explanation of the problem. Finally, systems practitioners warn against relying on archetypes too heavily.[21,22] In the *Fifth Discipline Fieldbook*, John Sterman, director of MIT System Dynamics Group, admits they are valuable as a first approach to understanding and revealing structure.[22] Yet, even with the simplest archetype he argues that predicting behavior means you are "trying to solve a high order non-linear differential equation in your head," which humans do not have the capacity to do. The purpose of including Sterman's comments is not to discourage the use of archetypes but to point to their limitations and emphasize that use of computer simulation modeling may be warranted in some situations.

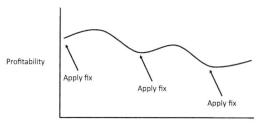

Fig. 7. Fixes that Backfire pattern of behavior. (*Adapted from* Goodman M. System archetypes. In: John B. Armstrong lectureship in systems thinking proceedings. Innovation Associates Organizational Learning. 2011;2(11):4.6; with permission.)

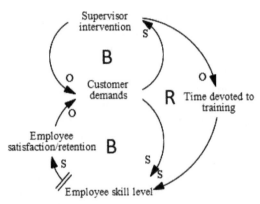

Fig. 8. Shifting the Burden archetype.

Mental Models

The final feature to identify are mental models, which are at the deepest level of structure. These are the assumptions and ideas we have about ourselves, others, our institutions, and how the world works.[9] They serve an important purpose because they help us make sense of complexity and we use them to reason and make decisions.[23] However, they are problematic as they are only simplified representations of reality[23] leading us to make to decisions based on incomplete information and incorrect assumptions.[24] Mental models exist at the individual and organizational levels and if not addressed will continue to affect system performance.[25]

The conversations surrounding mental models can be quite difficult at times. Individuals are asked to consider how their thoughts and assumptions contribute to problems[11] and strong emotions may emerge when it is discovered that actions and behaviors are a result of flawed assumptions.[26] Establishing a balance between discussion and dialogue early in the systems thinking process may make these and other conversations less difficult and improve overall learning.

Peter Senge specifically addresses this balance in *The Fifth Discipline*.[27] He suggests the purpose of discussion is to present and defend a point of view that is useful when analyzing the entirety of the situation or determining a course of action. However, in dialogue, the objective is to suspend our assumptions so we can explore the

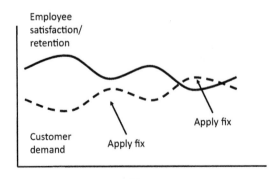

Fig. 9. Shifting the burden pattern of behavior.

unique thoughts of others and find the flaws in our own thinking. This creates an environment in which opinions are freely shared, individuals become more creative and less defensive and most important, collective learning occurs providing us with a deeper understanding of the issue.

Once mental models are revealed, they need to be included in system diagrams because of their influence. They are demonstrated in one of several ways: as a variable within a loop, the extent that a certain mental model is held, or as a thought bubble attached to an arrow between two variables.[12]

An example of a mental model that may exist in Fixes that Backfire (Figure 6) is "cost is the only thing I can control." This would have a powerful influence on decisions and may prevent the company from exploring other alternatives for managing their financial challenges. In Shifting the Burden (Figure 8), supervisors may have developed the mental model that "customer service is my most important role" as that is what they do most often. They may also receive recognition from their peers and upper management for their heroic efforts to save the company, thus further solidifying this notion.

Leverage Points/Interventions

The final step in systems thinking is identifying leverage points or interventions within the structure. This usually consists of one or two changes that will fundamentally improve the system yet minimize unintended consequences.[12]

In some cases, simply being aware of how the system functions can lead to different actions and behaviors.[11] Other strategies may be minimizing or eliminating time delays, rewiring of cause-and-effect relationships, shifting mental models, or aligning goals and metrics with chosen purpose.[11]

Some possible interventions in the Fixes that Backfire example may be

- Creating awareness of the impact of input reduction on production;
- Continuing to employ the input reduction strategy but in moderation to minimize the impact on production; and
- Further exploring possible causes of financial problems that input reductions were meant to fix.

In the Shifting the Burden example,

- Emphasize supervisor responsibilities and implement a system that rewards training instead of intervention.
- Use supervisor intervention as an opportunity to provide on-the-job training.
- Create awareness that the impact of the intervention will not be immediate and customer demand issues will likely worsen while supervisors are focused on training.

Once key leverage points have been identified, you can trace the impacts through your model to see if it has a positive impact long-term and look for possible unintended consequences.[12] As you might imagine, the real test will come with implementation and follow-up will be required to determine if it had the desired effect or if other interventions are necessary.

SUMMARY

At its surface, systems thinking appears to be a fairly simple process—describe events, trends, and patterns; reveal structure; then change the system. However, when applied to its fullest extent, it is a challenging, iterative process intermingled with periods of time where it feels like no progress is being made and finally a new view emerges.

Personal experience suggests that people exposed to systems thinking for the first time will generally fall into one of three categories: those who immediately see value and want more information, those who think there is value but not sure how it applies to them, and those who disregard it altogether.

To the individuals in the first category, a variety of resources have been referenced in this article, which will provide a good foundation and just like it is with any new skill, practice will be important. To those in the second category, other articles in this edition will provide examples of how systems thinking is being applied in veterinary medicine and agriculture and may provide insights on how it applies in your situation. Finally, for those in the third category, the suggestion is to keep an open mind. Even though you may not see value in applying each and every step, awareness of system behaviors may be all that is needed to gain a new perspective on an old problem.

INTEGRATION OF SYSTEMS THINKING IN RANCH MANAGEMENT (SIDE BAR)

Dr. Barry Dunn was first exposed to systems thinking during his PhD program at South Dakota State University. He had the opportunity to attend several workshops in both systems thinking and system dynamics, in which he interacted with thought leaders such as Michael Goodman, John Sterman, Nelson Repenning, and Jay Forrester. Those experiences had a profound effect on him and allowed him to move beyond just recognizing the complexity of systems to understanding it.

When Dr. Dunn was hired as the first Executive Director of King Ranch Institute for Ranch Management at Texas A&M–Kingsville in 2004, his vision was to create a program in which students were not only exposed to foundational topics in ranch management but also equipped to sort through the complexity of ranching instead of being paralyzed by it. As a result, he hired Michael Goodman to teach a systems thinking workshop, which became an annual event that has been attended by students, faculty, ranch managers/owners, and veterinarians from all over the United States. The workshops continue to this day but are led by a different instructor.

ACKNOWLEDGMENTS

Thank you to Michael Goodman for providing information that contributed to the section System Dynamics to Systems Thinking and Dr. Barry Dunn for providing information that contributed to the sidebar titled Integration of Systems Thinking in Ranch Management.

CONFLICTS OF INTEREST

The author has nothing to disclose.

REFERENCES

1. Ahn AC, Tewari M, Poon C-S, et al. The limits of reductionism in medicine: could systems biology offer an alternative? PLoS Med 2006;3(6):e208. Available at: https://doi.org/10.1371/journal.pmed.0030208. Accessed September 21, 2021.
2. Beresford MJ. Medical reductionism: lessons from the great philosophers. QJM 2010;103(9):721–4.
3. Kay J. An introduction to systems thinking. In: Waltner-Toews D, Kay JJ, editors. Lister NE. The ecosystem approach: complexity, uncertainty, and managing for sustainability. New York: Columbia University Press; 2008. p. 3–14.
4. Friedman B, Allen K. Systems theory. In: Brandell JR, editor. Essentials of clinical social work. Los Angeles: Sage Publications; 2014. p. 3–20.

5. Von Bertalnffy L. History and status of general systems theory. Acad Manage J 1972;15(4):407–26.
6. Ramage M, Shipp K. Introduction to the first edition. In: Systems thinking. 2nd edition. London: Springer; 2020. xii-xx.
7. Systems Dynamic Society webpage. 2021. Available at: https://systemdynamics.org/what-is-system-dynamics/. Accessed: September 2, 2021.
8. Meadows DH. The basics. In: Thinking in systems: a primer. White River Junction: Chelsea Publishing Company; 2008. p. 11–34.
9. Senge PM, Kleiner A, Roberts C, et al. The fifth discipline fieldbook: strategies and tools for building a learning organization. New York: Doubleday; 1994.
10. Forrester JW. The beginning of system dynamics. In: Banquet talk at the international systems dynamics society. 1989. Available at: https://web.mit.edu/sysdyn/sd-intro/D-4165-1.pdf. Accessed September 7, 2021.
11. Stroh DP. Systems thinking for social change. White River Junction: Chelsea Green Publishing; 2015.
12. Goodman M. In: John B. Armstrong lectureship in systems thinking proceeding. Innovation Associates organizational learning (version 02.11); 2011.
13. Goodman M, Immediato S. Applying systems thinking and common archetypes. 2006. Available at: https://www.iseesystems.com/store/training/applying-systems-thinking/. Accessed: September 14, 2021.
14. Kim D, Mullen E. The spirit of the learning organization. In: Systems thinker. 2018. Available at: https://thesystemsthinker.com/the-spirit-of-the-learning-organization/. Accessed: September 23, 2021.
15. Groves JT. Becoming indispensable by using systems thinking to tackle challenging and complex problems in practice. Am Assoc Bovine Pract Proc 2018; 51(2):111–2.
16. Goodman M, Kemeny J, Roberts C. The language of systems thinking: links and loop. In: Senge PM, Kleiner A, Roberts C, et al, editors. The fifth discipline fieldbook: strategies and tools for building a learning organization. New York: Doubleday; 1994. p. 113–48.
17. Wardman K. Anatomy of a reinforcing loop. In: Systems thinker. 2018. Available at: https://thesystemsthinker.com/anatomy-of-a-reinforcing-loop/. Accessed: September 7, 2021.
18. Levy M, Tasoff J. Exponential growth bias and overconfidence. J Econ Psychol 2017;58:1–14.
19. Herasymowych M, Senko H. Positive systems archetypes. In: Systems thinker. 2018. Available at: https://thesystemsthinker.com/positive-systems-archetypes/. Accessed: September 10, 2021.
20. Kim DH, Anderson V. Shifting the burden. In: Systems archetype basics: from story to structure. Westford: Pegasus Communications. 2011. 2021. p. 25–41. Available at: https://thesystemsthinker.com/wp-content/uploads/2016/03/Systems-Archetypes-Basics-WB002E.pdf. Accessed: September 10, 2021.
21. Fisher LM. The prophet of unintended consequences. In: Strategy + business. 2005. Available at: https://www.strategy-business.com/article/05308?pg=0. Accessed August 10, 2021.
22. Sterman J. Beyond training wheels. In: Senge PM, Kleiner A, Roberts C, et al, editors. The fifth discipline fieldbook: strategies and tools for building a learning organization. New York: Doubleday; 1994. p. 177–84.
23. Jones NA, Ross H, Lynam T, et al. Mental models: an interdisciplinary synthesis of theory and methods. Ecol Soc 2011;16(1):46. Available at: http://www.ecologyandsociety.org/vol16/iss1/art46/. Accessed: September 22, 2021.

24. World Bank. Thinking with mental models. In: World development report 2015: mind, society, and behavior. Washington, DC: World Bank; 2015. p. 62–75. Available at: https://ccsi.org/CCSI/media/pdfs/DAY1_Chapter-3_Thinking_with_Mental_Models.pdf. Accessed: September 24, 2021.
25. Magzan M. Mental models for leadership effectiveness: building future different than the past. JEMC 2012;2(2):57–63.
26. Roberts C. What you can expect when working with mental models. In: Senge PM, Kleiner A, Roberts C, et al, editors. The fifth discipline fieldbook: strategies and tools for building a learning organization. New York: Doubleday; 1994. p. 239–42.
27. Senge PM. The fifth discipline: the art and practice of a learning organization. revised edition. New York: Crown Business; 2006.

Beef Production Health Systems

Perspectives of a Trained Systems Thinker

Benjamin L. Turner, PhD*

KEYWORDS

- Morbidity • Integrated beef production • System dynamics • Mental models

KEY POINTS

- Understanding and working with mental models is a critical part of the systems thinking process.
- System dynamics models provide means to explore feedback-rich problems in cost-effective ways where reductionistic methods often fall short.
- Mental models of beef production stakeholders possess a high degree of leverage over production performance but have often gone underappreciated.

INTRODUCTION

Throughout this article, a foundation is established that differentiates the systems thinking approach from our traditionally trained reductionist forms of thinking. Numerous examples have been given where the "status quo" approach to management failed or perhaps made problems even worse. Despite all that we know about the limitations of the "status quo" thinking in light of the complex, dynamic systems we are embedded in, why do scientists and managers continue to rely on old habits of thought? Why is sustainable change and innovation not "the norm" across sectors of the beef production system rather than the exception?

Following the systems thinking process outlined by Payne,[1] this article sets out to explore the role of mental models. Mental models are deep-rooted elements of systemic structure often responsible for either perpetuating problematic behavior patterns or leading the way out of them. To examine the influence of mental models underlying beef production health problems, we examine 2 case studies through systems-oriented lenses:

Associate Professor, Department of Agriculture, Agribusiness, and Environmental Science and King Ranch Institute for Ranch Management, Texas A&M University-Kingsville, 700 University Boulevard MSC 228, Kingsville, TX 78636, USA
* Corresponding author.
E-mail address: benjamin.turner@tamuk.edu

Vet Clin Food Anim 38 (2022) 179–200
https://doi.org/10.1016/j.cvfa.2022.02.005
0749-0720/22/© 2022 Elsevier Inc. All rights reserved.
vetfood.theclinics.com

- The increase in industry-wide morbidity problems, using the Iceberg Diagram process
- The morbidity crisis in a single, integrated beef production organization, using system dynamics modeling

After presenting each case, we discuss the powerful role of mental models involved in each problem, developing clear, articulatable, and feedback-based descriptions of how mental models created and interacted with other structural elements to contribute to the problem at hand.

PERSISTENT MORBIDITY IN THE BEEF SUPPLY CHAIN
Visualizing the Iceberg Diagram Process

The first step in the systems thinking process is having a clearly defined and articulated problem. In this case, the problem we want to understand more clearly at a deeper, structural level is the persistent morbidity of calves in the beef cattle production and marketing system. Morbidity is most often managed through medical treatment, which reduces the bottom line in the form of greater chemical inputs and labor and less revenues due to losses in productivity.[2-4] Mortality and morbidity rates are closely correlated (ie, livestock with greater than average medical treatment costs have higher-than-average mortality rates[5,6]). Interestingly, processing costs (ie, the time, labor, and energy needed to receive, treat, process, and ship) are also closely correlated to mortality rates.[5,6] Increased mortality rates mean fewer animals to market and therefore fewer revenue-generating animals to cover the costs of the entire animal population, creating a longer-term economic stress to the production system. These issues are particularly chronic in the feeding sector of the industry.[7-11] Looking at the issue through a systems thinking lens, we may ask ourselves, "Despite improved understanding of bovine vaccine potential and state-of-the-art management technology, why does the beef industry continue to struggle with rising post-weaning morbidity and mortality?" To gain a deeper understanding of the morbidity problem, we follow the systems thinking process down from the event to the structural level (see the Iceberg Diagram in the article by Payne[1]). The top of the Iceberg Diagram begins with the perception of a major outbreak or "spike" in morbidity rate that seems to be out of the ordinary. As a major event, it forces us to react in the short term. But as systems thinkers, it should pique our curiosity to "dig deeper" and understand why such an outbreak occurs to change the way we manage our reactions and strategies moving forward. With our curiosity engaged, we can look down the iceberg, through Trends and Structure, so that we can better manage the structure of the problem and create a situation in which events, such as morbidity "spikes," occur less often and with less severity.

There are several key trends and behavior patterns one can observe to better understand how the beef industry has evolved over time and what those changes mean for beef animal health, including but not limited to the following:

- Morbidity rate: obviously, if we want better management of morbidity, we should understand how it has changed over time, as the famous business adage warns: "you can't manage what you don't measure." Over time, we have observed morbidity rates increasing[9,12] (**Fig. 1**A).
- Mortality rate: mortality rates have risen with rising morbidity[9,10,12,13] (**Fig. 1**B).
- Costs: cost of time, labor, and medical treatments continue to increase, a function of both beef morbidity and market costs[14] (**Fig. 1**C). Ranch-level costs also continue to increase at the cow-calf level[15] (**Fig. 1**D).

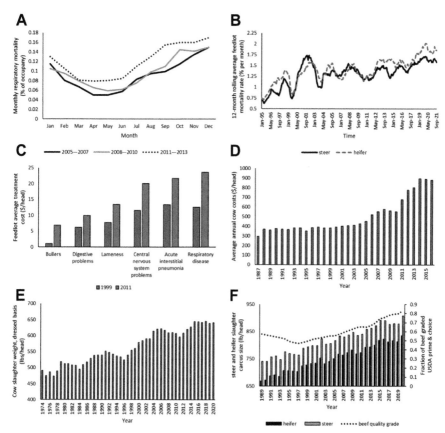

Fig. 1. Trends and patterns over time relevant to the beef morbidity problem: increased incidence of BRD9 (*A*); increased mortality rates of steers and heifers[13] (*B*); increased costs of feedlot health treatments[14] (*C*), and on-ranch cow costs (*D*); increasing cow slaughter weight used as a proxy for cow size (*E*), and increased steer and heifer slaughter carcass sizes[16] and quality grades[18] (*F*).

- Selection for growth traits: with costs increasing, lost production potential due to morbidity and mortality, and constraints on management, labor, and inputs, the cattle industry has continued to prioritize growth potential in the US herd. Producers have responded via greater breeding selection that maximizes growth (ie, carcass sizes and by default, cow sizes)[16] and quality[17,18] in an attempt to maximize returns (**Fig. 1**E).
- Demand for animal welfare: with greater consumer sensitivity to climate, environmental, and food system problems, demand for documented efforts to enhance animal welfare before harvest continues to increase.[17]

In terms of structure, there are several critical elements of physical, socioeconomic, industry, and personal (mental model) structures that give rise to and create the trends and patterns observed over time:

- Biophysical structure: Physically, the US beef cattle industry is geographically dispersed across all 50 states, with cattle operations in environments ranging from coastal to montane ecosystems and arid to tropical climate regimes. Because of this, livestock for feeding are sourced nationwide and over all parts of the year. Several regions are especially critical for the US beef supply, particularly the Great Plains, western, and southwestern regions. In addition, the biological nature of production (ie, animal- and plant-based production systems) creates a plethora of growth, health, and economic constraints.

- Industry structure: The US beef cattle industry remains a horizontally integrated supply chain, where stakeholders at each stage of the supply process are stand-alone enterprises, with little to no integration with preproduction or postproduction stages (ie, little integration between cow-calf, stocker, feedlot/finishing, and packing sectors). However, there has been considerable consolidation within sectors, meaning that there are fewer and fewer, but larger and larger, enterprises operating in a given sector, with consolidation being most pronounced at the packer and finishing stages and less pronounced at the cow-calf and stocker stages. In addition, these sectors are geographically distinct: the feeding and packing sectors are heavily concentrated in the western plains states such as Texas, Oklahoma, and Colorado; the stocker sector is seasonally distributed along central plains north and south; and the cow-calf sector is more evenly distributed across the nation depending on how well climate and ecosystem characteristics provide adequate forage and water supply to support grazing animals. This fact influences when calves progress through the supply chain (eg, fall- vs spring-weaned calves), how prepared they are to perform in a new environment (eg, preconditioned or not), and how at-risk calves are contracting diseases (eg, marketed lots of similar age, size, genetics, and source ranch vs commingled cattle with diverse features from multiple ranches).

- Socioeconomic structure: Given the highly segmented, dis-integrated nature of beef production enterprises throughout the supply chain, differing socioeconomic goals and constraints, such as those dealing with profitability, family business transition, lifestyle, shareholder wealth, consumer satisfaction and perception, among many others, provide discontinuous incentives to producers depending on which sector they operate in. For example, it is reasonable for cow-calf production to maximize profitability at the cow-calf level, even if that means reduced returns for stockers or feeders. Likewise, efforts by the packing industry to maximize profitability have led that sector to exert strong price pressure on the other industry sectors; this is also reinforced given the industry structure of consolidation, which gives increasing market power to those sectors that have coalesced capital and resources to the fewest number of enterprises. Results from these types of decisions have an array of unintended, feedback reinforcing consequences on industry trends and events.

Because of the aforementioned structural considerations, cattle move through a complex production and marketing system, often through multiple handling and processing facilities (eg, auctions), beginning as early as the time of weaning when calf immune systems are still immature.[10] Given these "big picture" structures of the beef production industry, what specific structures converge that contribute to the escalating beef morbidity problem?

- Genetic focus in beef cattle breeding regimes, "you can't manage what you don't measure": With greater emphasis on growth potential and genetic traits conducive to weaning weight, calving ease, and marbling, other important and economically valubale genetic traits useful for minimizing health risk remain unexplored. More dynamically, when monitoring and performance data collection are designed around existing expected progeny difference (EPD) metrics, use of those metrics is reinforced, and opportunities are minimized to identify, measure, and index the interaction of varying traits and their genetic markers that would be useful for developing indexes balancing performance and health, which in general is lacking in the beef industry relative to other important livestock species.[19]

- Probability of preweaning vaccination and incentives to do so: Surveys have indicated that as many as 61% of beef cattle producers do not vaccinate for respiratory disease, which may be as high as 74% for operations with fewer than 50 mature cows.[10,20] Conversely, producers of 200 or more head that do not vaccinate for respiratory disease is as low as 18%. Industry wide, about 70% of all calves are administered respiratory vaccinations, whereas 30% are not, and only 25% of all beef cow operations vaccinate for each of the common respiratory viruses infectious bovine rhinotracheitis virus (IBRV), bovine viral diarrhea virus (BVDV), parainfluenza 3 (PI3V), or bovine respiratory syncytial virus (BRSV).[10,20] This discrepancy between large and small operations is likely exacerbated by economic incentives: larger operations more likely to fulfill order buyer or contractor specifications for large, uniform lots of calves for a premium can see a return on investment in vaccination implementation, whereas smaller producers supplying a few numbers of calves are less likely to meet such specifications for a premium and therefore fail to invest in vaccinations.

- Geographic distance to finishing and commingling effects: Consolidation of the feeding and packing industry into a few operations in the southwestern and western United States means that shipping times and distances that calves must endure to reach the feedlot are, on average, longer than in previous decades. As the cow-calf sector evolves toward fewer, larger ranches, resulting in a small number of ranches supplying a disproportionately large percentage of all calves produced, large-scale producers are more apt to take advantage of pricing signals for calf health treatments (see previous point). Total calf production will not be affected by such consolidation at the cow-calf level, but the timing of events through the system may be altered because larger operations are more likely to follow tightly defined breeding and calving seasons and weaning protocols. Downstream buyers, to maintain cattle flows between supply surges, have to fill more lots with commingled cattle that originate from smaller producers. Although producers with 50 head or less supply a relatively small fraction of the total calves to the system, the risk effect of nonvaccination is compounded as their calves are forced to become commingled together as they mature through the system.

- Mental model or personal structure: How do we as individuals respond to and interact with the biophysical, industrial, and socioeconomic structures described earlier? What are some common voices one may hear when listening to managers on the ground? These voices that echo the decision-making goals, values, beliefs, and assumptions vary by sector across the industry and by region across the country. Regardless of where we are, however, we often hear voices such as "We can't see a return for our investment" when considering investment in the time, labor, and resources for vaccination (cow-calf); "If I don't commingle some lots together I won't have the volume I need later" (stocker); and "If we just get these lots through the first few days we'll be in the clear" or "Continued treatment can't possibly hurt," so long as the problem is handled now, in the short-term, to bring performance levels back to the perceived level of its potential (feedyard).

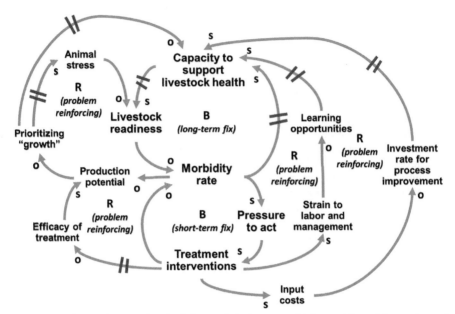

Fig. 2. Causal loop diagram (CLD) of the cattle industry morbidity problem. All notations of Ss, Os, Rs, and Bs follow the convention of feedback links and loops outlined by Payne[1] in this article. Note that the CLD in composed of both short- and long-term intervention strategies, but due to the unintended consequences of short-term vaccination treatments, the problem is made worse in the long-term ("Fixes that Backfires," 2 bottom left R loops) or make it more difficult and costly to implement long-term solutions (a "Shifting the Burden" archetype, 2 outer R loops at right).

Archetype Development

After identifying important trends and patterns over time and then thinking deeply about the underlying structure that can account for such behaviors, we are liable to find still additional complexity not captured in the current Iceberg Diagram. However, there are some components that we can start to connect into reinforcing and balancing feedback processes to give ourselves a glimpse into the deeper structural forces that perpetuate beef cattle morbidity over time (**Fig. 2**). Starting with morbidity rate as the core problem of interest, we can infer there are both short- and long-term solutions (balancing processes) that will offset the problem and reduce morbidity: intervene with traditional medical treatment (labeled "short-term fix" in **Fig. 2**) or improve the capacity to support livestock health and therefore livestock readiness to combat disease or illness (labeled "long-term fix" in **Fig. 2**). Most often today, we are relying on the "short-term fix" of medical treatment. Unfortunately, there are an array of unintended consequences (biophysical, economic, and personal) to that strategy and impede our ability to use the long-term fix.

Biophysically, as the reliance on treatment interventions grows, the efficacy of treatment is eventually eroded (after some time delay), which comes back to reinforce the morbidity rate when conditions are right for it. Economically, treatment costs are significant. The increased input costs in time, labor, vaccinations, and implicit costs erode the potential investment rate for process improvement. Without longer-term investment to develop and implement improved management processes and practices, the capacity to support livestock health is constrained. From a personnel management perspective, relying on the short-term fix creates strain to labor and management that minimizes opportunities for learning and growth that is needed to formulate creative and innovative ways to adapt production processes to be more conducive to supporting livestock health. As morbidity increases and the efficacy of treatment diminishes, the ability of the animal to meet its production potential wanes. In an attempt to restore lost productivity, the message to prioritize growth (via market price signals) feeds back to the cow-calf sector, which has responded to those signals via breeding programs designed to maximize weaning weights and carcass characteristics. Such investment has taken away from other possible investments in capacity to support livestock health (eg, preconditioning or backgrounding facilities and expertise, developing multitrait selection indices for profitability, which include leading indicators of health risk) and added to overall animal stress given the acceleration in growth rates and unintended consequence of worsened crowding in transport given overall increase in animal size. The less ready and able the animal is to perform due to such stresses, the more likely it is to suffer from disease in the finishing stage. All of these unintended consequences reinforce the reliance on the short-term fix (treatment interventions), meaning we only address the symptoms of morbidity and not the underlying structural causes.

The archetype structure shown in **Fig. 2** includes several Fixes that Backfire[21,22] (the problem reinforcing loops on the bottom left and top left, both of which are coupled to the central variable, morbidity rate) and Shifting the Burden[21,22] (the 2 problem reinforcing loops on the right that couple together the short-term fix, treatment interventions, with the long-term alternative, building capacity to support livestock health).

UNEXPECTED DISEASE OUTBREAK IN AN INTEGRATED BEEF PRODUCTION SYSTEM
Background

A rancher-owned integrated beef company (birth to packing) headquartered in a western US state sources calves from ranches throughout the American west and southwest. One of the goals of the company is to link production operations directly to retail beef consumers through an "all-natural" beef product that is traceable from the retail counter to the home ranch. The process is certified by third-party auditors that ensure cattle are raised humanely (eg, never fed animal-derived feedstuffs or given antibiotics or hormones). Doing so allows the company to supply cattle to a niche beef retail market. Morbid animals that do receive therapeutic antibiotics fail to qualify for the niche market; consequently, treated animals are removed from niche program sales and are sold on the conventional beef market (called "out-of-program" calves).

During the third quarter last year, the number of "out-of-program" calves having receiving antibiotic treatment for morbidity dramatically increased, up to 7.3%, compared with its historic expected average of 2.4%. This increase likewise escalated production costs to the point of potential disruption of the ability to continue flowing cattle through the system. With fewer calves qualifying for the niche program, the company was jeopardized in not being able to supply its expected retail demand. In response, upper management began an internal investigation to identify the causes of the morbidity "spike" and the cattle health-related risk factors that contributed to it.

Investigating Trends and Patterns and Organizational Structure

Any available data that could inform management about the problem were pulled together to examine the situation in more detail, be it from the home ranches, feedlot, or the accountant's office. What they discovered alarmed them. Over the previous 5 years, mean morbidity rates (expressed percent of occupancy at month of

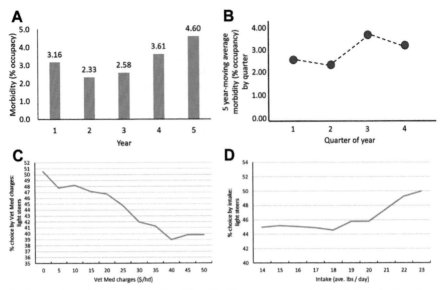

Fig. 3. Trends and patterns over time identified by management of the integrated beef supply company to better understand their feedlot morbidity crisis: mean morbidity over previous 5-year period (A), mean morbidity rate by quarter (B), percent of steer carcasses graded choice as a function of veterinary treatment costs (C), and percent of steer carcasses graded choice as a function of average daily intake (D). (All data provided by Dunn BH. 2009. Unpublished data. King Ranch Institute for Ranch Management, Texas A&M University, Kingsville.)

occurrence) had climbed to nearly 5% (**Fig. 3**A) and were worst during the third quarter of the year (see **Fig. 3**B), a time when industry averages are less than the first or fourth quarters (compared with Vogel and colleagues[9]). Data from closeouts indicated that carcass quality was negatively affected by veterinary treatment costs (a proxy for severity of morbidity), whereas positively correlated with intake (see **Fig. 3**D), assuming morbid animals reduce intake. The quality of calves entering the system was very good, a testament to the member ranchers supplying calves to the program, and no major morbidity crises were observed at home ranches, although some believed newer members forced to place calves in winter or those ranches farther away geographically could have been the source of the concern. After careful deliberation and consideration of the facts, management determined that morbidity trends were indeed worsening and not enough was being done at the feedlot to ensure calf health and performance.

Management Response and Consequences

After their investigation, management created a livestock insurance program aimed at the feedlot, where increasing morbidity was dramatically eroding financial returns through the escalation of "out-of-program" beef sales. The intended strategy was to alleviate financial pressure through increasing feedlot capacity to be able feed and finish increased numbers of conventional cattle sold on the conventional market. To achieve this, ownership purchased additional livestock from nonmember ranchers (called "insurance calves") to finish in feedlot pens newly designated for only insurance calves and sale as "out-of-program" beef on the conventional market. The new supplemental revenue stream generated from these conventional beef sales was then redistributed to member ranches to compensate for premium losses of owned cattle as a result of feedlot morbidity issues.

Although initially deemed a success, it did not take long before the company thought it needed to go "back to the drawing board." Expanding the "out-of-program" livestock placed additional stress on the feedlot. Managers were now running 2 feeding enterprises instead of one, with different processing procedures, feed sources, record keeping requirements, and supplier relationships. Insurance calves may arrive as uniform lots from single sources or highly commingled lots from multiple sources. Given space constraints, maintaining adequate separation between in-program and insurance calves became more problematic. As a result, minimizing morbidity became more challenging instead of less, and with more financial resources being used to support the new revenue stream, the margin for error for in-program practices shrunk. More subtly, member ranchers' perceptions of in-program premium protection was elevated due to the implementation of the "insurance calves" strategy, and therefore investments in ranch-level efforts to improve animal health were redirected to other concerns on ranch, undermining efforts to curtail morbidity risk of calves entering the feedlot.

The feedback structure of the morbidity problem, management response, and unintended consequences are shown in the causal loop diagram in **Fig. 4.**

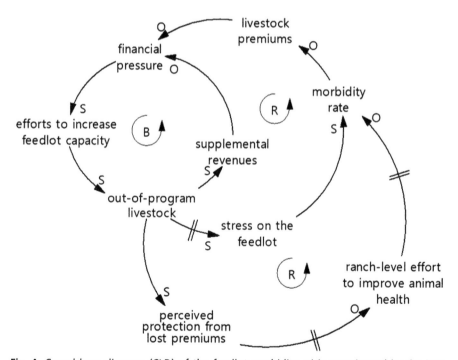

Fig. 4. Causal loop diagram (CLD) of the feedlot morbidity crisis experienced by the integrated beef supply company. All notations of Ss, Os, Rs, and Bs follow the convention of feedback links and loops outlined by Payne[1] in this article. In this case, the problem of morbidity rate was addressed financially by increasing feeding capacity and out-of-program production (balancing loop at left, a short-term fix) whose unintended consequences of stress to the feedlot and perceived protection to contributing ranchers masked problems of calf readiness to finish and actually reinforced morbidity rate problems rather than mitigate it (top and bottom reinforcing loops at right).

Stock-and-Flow Feedback Model

After unsuccessful implementation of the insurance strategy, management reached out to several external beef industry consultants. After studying the issue, one consultant group, trained in systems thinking and system dynamics modeling, translated the aforementioned causal loop diagram into a stock-and-flow model capable of mathematical simulation (stocks represent accumulations of material or information and can only change via flows, or rates of change over time, coupled via reinforcing and balancing feedback loops).[23] The simplified model, illustrated in **Fig. 5** and documented in **Table 1**, is described as follows.

Ranch A has an inflow and outflow of herd adjustments (expanding or shrinking herd size); this drives the number of eligible calves into the program from Ranch A.

Feedlot A, the core stock of the model, has an inflow of placements A (calves) that are driven by the eligible calves from Ranch A and arriving at the feedlot in the placement month. Feedlot A has 2 outflows. The first is harvest A (harvested "in-program" calves from feedlot), which occurs at the harvest month and includes all calves in Feedlot A not treated for morbidity issues. The second outflow is nonprogram calves, which include all calves treated for morbidity issues. Cumulative financial return is the financial stock, driven by the inflows of annual revenues (in-program calf price times the number of annual calves fulfilling the program plus any out-of-program revenue) and outflows (all costs associated with production, including costs to weaning at the ranch level plus finishing and treatment costs at the feedlot).

This structure is replicated for all other ranches, B, C, D, and so on, until all ranches were represented. The model includes a stock of cumulative in-program calves

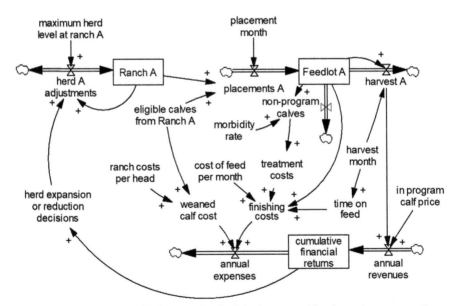

Fig. 5. Stock and flow model diagram (SFD) of the integrated beef supply company. Boxes represent stocks (or accumulations), thick black-and-white arrows represent flows (or the rates of change into or out of a stock), and thin blue arrows represent information feedback links. Here, positive notations stand for positive or reinforcing influence (similar to "S" in a CLD), whereas negative notations stand for negative or balancing influence (similar to "O" in a CLD).[23]

Table 1
Overview of simulation model equations

Variable	Equation	Unit	Type
Annual expenses	IF THEN ELSE (month counter = harvest month, weaned calf cost + finishing costs, 0)	$/Month	Flow
Annual revenues	IF THEN ELSE (month counter = harvest month, harvest A*in program calf price, 0)	$/Month	Flow
Cost of feed per month	375	$/hd/month	Auxiliary /Information
Cumulative financial returns	INTEG (annual revenues−annual expenses, 0)	$	Stock
Time on feed	(Harvest month−placement month)/month conversion	1	Auxiliary/ information
Eligible calves from Ranch A	0.9	1/Month	Auxiliary /information
Feedyard A	INTEG (placements A-harvest A-"nonprogram calves," 0)	hd	Stock
Finishing costs	(Feedyard A*days on feed*cost of feed per day)+treatment costs	$/Month	Auxiliary/ information
Harvest A	IF THEN ELSE (month counter = harvest month, Feedyard A/mo conversion*(1-morbidity rate), 0)	hd/Month	Flow
Harvest month	9	Month	Auxiliary/ information
Herd A adjustments	IF THEN ELSE (Ranch A > maximum herd level at ranch A, 0, IF THEN ELSE (Ranch A < maximum herd level at ranch A:AND: (Ranch A*herd expansion or reduction decisions)<(maximum herd level at Ranch A -Ranch A), (Ranch A*herd expansion or reduction decisions)/TIME STEP, ((Ranch A*herd expansion or reduction decisions)*(1-(Ranch A/maximum herd level at ranch A)))/TIME STEP))	hd/Month	Flow
Herd expansion or reduction decisions	WITH LOOKUP (cumulative financial returns, ([(0,0)-(1e+06,0.1)],(0,0),(1e+06,0)))	1/Month	Auxiliary/ information
Initial Ranch A herd size	500	hd	Auxiliary/ information
In-program calf price	2400	$/hd	Auxiliary/ information
Maximum herd level at ranch A	1000	hd	Auxiliary/ information

(continued on next page)

Table 1 (continued)			
Variable	**Equation**	**Unit**	**Type**
Month conversion	1	Month	Auxiliary/ information
Month counter	MODULO (Time, 12)	Month	Auxiliary/ information
Morbidity rate	0.15	1/Month	Auxiliary/ information
Nonprogram calves	IF THEN ELSE(harvest A>0, Feedyard A/month conversion- harvest A, 0)	hd/Month	Flow
Placement month	4	Month	Auxiliary/ Information
Placements A	IF THEN ELSE(month counter = placement month, Ranch A*eligible calves from Ranch A, 0)	hd/Month	Flow
Ranch A	INTEG (herd A adjustments, initial Ranch A herd size)	hd	Stock
Ranch costs per head	625	$/hd	Auxiliary/ information
TIME STEP	1	Month	Auxiliary/ information
Treatment cost per head	100	$/hd	Auxiliary/ information
Treatment costs	Nonprogram calves*treatment cost per head	$/Month	Auxiliary/ information
Weaned calf cost	(Ranch A*eligible calves from Ranch A)*ranch costs per head	$/Month	Auxiliary/ information

Conditional statements using IF THEN ELSE are translated as IF (condition met?) THEN (operation if true) ELSE (operation if false). INTEG represent stocks using mathematical integration over time, LOOKUP represents a dynamic table function where the variable looked up is the input used to determine a corresponding output variable used elsewhere in the model. MODULO represents a repeated time counter (in this case repeating every 12 months to track month of year). Time variables are model constants. Animal head is abbreviated as "hd" for simplicity.

(originating from all ranches), cumulative out-of-program calves (the annual number of calves treated for morbidity and marketed as out-of-program plus the number of "insurance calves" finished), and cumulative financial returns to the system (integrating the cumulative financial flows from all costs and sales).

The simulation model allowed the team to develop and test "what-if" scenarios to identify strategies currently eluding management that would lead to longer-term improvements in health performance and therefore profitability. The team hypothesized that a more sustainably profitable approach would be implementing a preconditioning program for all calves at the ranch level and any morbidity costs occurring at the feedlot to be billed to the ranch of origin.

Simulation Results

The simplified simulation model was run using the implemented fed cattle insurance program used by management and the hypothesized preconditioning practice for comparison over a 10-year evaluation period to compare cumulative in- and out-of-program

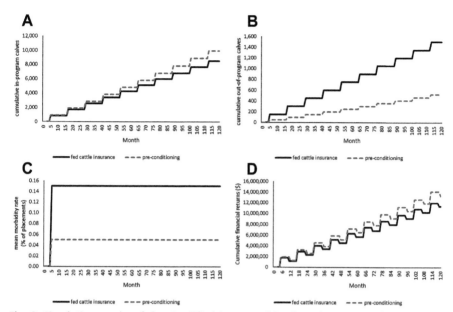

Fig. 6. Simulation results of the simplified integrated beef production supply chain, illustrating significant differences in number of in-program (*A*) and out-of-program (*B*) calves, mean morbidity rates (*C*), and cumulative financial return (*D*) given the insurance program or on-ranch preconditioning.

calves finished, mean morbidity rates, and cumulative financial returns. Results indicated that the preconditioning program would finish more than 1400 more in-program calves (**Fig. 6**A) and result in 1000 fewer out-of-program calves (see **Fig. 6**B), rendering the insurance program obsolete. The reason for this was the dramatic reduction in mean morbidity rates in member-owned calves under the preconditioning scenario as calves were better prepared and therefore less at risk for morbidity and treatment and being sold as out-of-program conventional beef (see **Fig. 6**C). The net result was a 17% increase in cumulative returns (see **Fig. 6**E).

THE POWER OF MENTAL MODELS
Mental Models Defined

Mental models represent the relationships and assumptions about a system held in a person's mind. A formal definition of mental model has been synthesized as "a relatively enduring and accessible, but limited, internal conceptual representation of a system (historic, existing, or projected) whose structure is analogous to the perceived structure of that system."[24] Mental models affect how we think and direct our actions. Some mental models may be conscious to us, while some may be embedded subconsciously. Often, it is easier to recognize others' mental models than to be able to describe our own. Importantly, mental models are always incomplete due to the limited processing and storage capacity of the human brain. Because of these limitations, we often craft mental "heuristics" (shortcuts or "rules of thumb") to better cope with the complexity and uncertainty around us.[25] If we are not careful, however, these mental shortcuts can reinforce our own mental model of a system, which if wrong, inaccurate, or biased, will perpetuate poor performance or negative unintended consequences. To illustrate how mental models reinforce themselves in such a way despite the undesirable

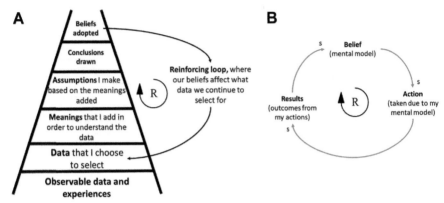

Fig. 7. Template of The Ladder of Inference in diagram form (*A*) and causal loop diagram (CLD) form (*B*). The CLD links can be read as 3 successive "S" links: as my belief template is strengthened, the actions I take remain on the same trajectory and I may even "double down" on those actions, the outcomes of which only become more pervasive because I did not change any actions, and as those outcomes appear I select data that only strengthens my original mental model.

outcomes, we turn to a concept just as elegant and perhaps more powerful than the Iceberg Diagram: The Ladder of Inference.[21]

The Ladder of Inference: the Source of Strength for Mental Models

Like the Iceberg Diagram helps us identify the structure underlying the surface of a particular problem, The Ladder of Inference helps us identify how and why particular mental models are reinforced. The Ladder of Inference, depicted in **Fig. 7**A, illustrates the process by which we build inferences about particular phenomena based on our real-life experiences and all the observable data available to us. Because we are limited in time, resources, and mental capacity, we select only a fraction of the available data and experience that we have access to, and from that reduced dataset we add meanings and build assumptions needed to draw our own conclusions. Based on the conclusions, both in thought and action, we shape our particular belief template. As we continue to confront new or evolving problems, rather than seek out the new and best available data, we select only those data that conform to our particular beliefs, thereby reinforcing the original belief. Over time, the beliefs, assumptions, and meanings about our experiences became ingrained. This process of reinforcing mental models and beliefs can be translated into a causal loop diagram (shown in **Fig. 7**B). Here, our beliefs lead us to particular actions, those actions create particular outcomes, and we select data from those outcomes (perceived or real) that reinforce our original belief.

Belief-Action-Results Loops Underlying Beef Morbidity Crises

Having made the foundations of mental models explicit in the previous section using The Ladder of Inference, now we revisit 2 case studies: industry-wide morbidity problems and unexpected outbreaks in integrated beef production systems. To summarize, the pervasive mental models observed or expressed by stakeholders could be described in the following:

- Industry-wide morbidity: At the cow-calf level, many producers, especially those small-scale operations marketing fewer than 50 head, are resigned to any vaccination program, "We can't see a return for our investment." Meanwhile, the stocker segment, especially squeezed on the financial margins at both ends, does not have the time or incentive to look for new ways of doing things, because "if I don't get the volume I need [via comingling] I'm not going to be in business next year." Finally, the feedlots, who integrate the entire morbidity problem in one place because they are where all cattle eventually flow, have to have immediate solutions to get cattle back on feed, otherwise the entire system stalls. "Continued treatment can't possibly hurt… especially early, if we just get new lots through the first few days we'll be in the clear."

- Integrated beef production system: Management of the system held the feedlot responsible for the morbidity crisis. "Cattle were not sick on their home ranches, which are some of the best in the country… the alarming trend is isolated to the feedlot, that is where change will be most effective."

If the deepest part of the iceberg's structure is our own mental models, and the power of mental models is created by the reinforcing nature by which we select and use only those data that support our beliefs, what subtle processes might be at work below the level of our awareness that reinforce these mental models? To answer that question, we have to look at what data or observations *have not* been selected for, either now or in the past, and therefore have eluded our thought formation process relative to the data that we have selected for. As the old adage goes, "It ain't what you don't know that gets you in trouble, it's what you know for sure that just ain't so."

In the industry-wide case, a prevailing mental model at the feedlot sector pertains to widespread (metaphylactic) antimicrobial treatment practices either on arrival or within a few days during initial processing procedures when stress is greatest,[8,26] which is grounded in the evidence that the first 42 to 45 days on feed represent the most significant risk of disease onset, particularly bovine respiratory disease (BRD), which negatively affects performance.[27–29] Besides performance, widespread metaphylactic antimicrobial treatment is also a preferable risk management tool given it not only reduces individual cases but also may reduce the risk of pen-level disease by limiting its spread in the environment.[8] Data that have not been selected for in the development of feedlot management "rules of thumb" include evidence that health risk is more uniform throughout feeding period than originally expected[9,11] (especially for high-performing calves)[11] and that metaphylactic treatment delays visual feedback on which animals need therapy,[28] the interaction of which means that "mortality is not isolated to the receiving period and occurs at comparable rates thereafter"[9] (**Fig. 8**A). The impact on performance means that the cumulative number of calves affected by morbidity does not stabilize after initial treatment but is more likely to continue increasing with days on feed (see **Fig. 8**B).

If there are good data that would lead one to revisit the feedlot "rule of thumb" for early widespread vaccination, why has the practice been so slow to be updated? The belief-action-result loop may help unravel why (see **Fig. 8**C). Given the mental model belief that "If we just get these lots [of calves] through the first few days we'll be in the clear," actions are taken aimed at widespread early treatment in hopes of prevention. Because of this, less attention to the problem is paid over time as days on feeding increases. Such behavior leads to some expected results. Initial calves needing and receiving treatment "make it." However, unintended results, such as problem calves experiencing delayed onset (and potentially high performers), are less likely to be treated when they actually need it (i.e., mismatching onset of disease with treatment time). With reduced performance or rising calf losses, management

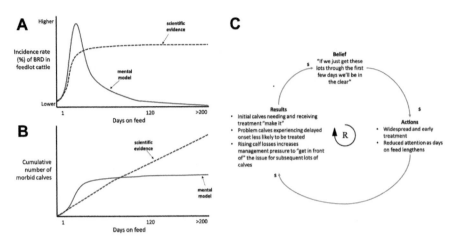

Fig. 8. Mental model inferences regarding calf morbidity risk and its effect on reinforcing existing beliefs: inferred incidence rate of BRD compared with existing evidence[9,11] (*A*) and the resultant expectation regarding cumulative numbers of calves experiencing morbidity (*B*), both of which contribute to the reinforcing belief-action-result process that engrains the original mental model (*C*).

pressure mounts to "get in front of" the issue for subsequent lots of calves, reinforcing early and widespread vaccination.

The mental model dynamics of the integrated beef production operation expressed itself a bit differently but just as powerfully. Management perceived a trend in feedlot morbidity due to selection effects in the data for several reasons. First, the aggregate feedlot data suggested cattle were performing as expected given they were subject to treatment or not, which conformed to their expectations about feedlot management (see **Fig. 3**). Second, cattle were not sick on home ranches and neither did partner ranches want to blame themselves or their peers for causing or contributing to the issue. Data that were not selected for but were readily available to management dealt with home ranch characteristics and how those influenced feedlot performance (**Fig. 9**). For example, home ranches were located throughout the west in extremely varied environmental and ecological conditions necessitating ranch operations fit to individual, unique environments (see **Fig. 9**A). Ranches were also not uniformly distanced from the feedlot, and this meant that placements were arriving at different times of the year with very different stress levels and readiness to perform, which was reflected in the individual lot performance data. Although the mean quality grades seemed reasonable to management, individual lots told a different story. The percentage of steers grading choice was nearly independent of veterinary medical costs (see **Fig. 9**B) or average daily intake (see **Fig. 9**C). Such variability indicated that morbidity was more likely a function of individual lot assignment, itself a function of ranch of origin. In short, management failed to appropriately account for factors outside of the feedlot as sources of the crisis.

If these data were available, what made it so difficult to internalize for management and the home ranches who had invested in the company? Here again the belief-action-result loop helps paint a rich picture of the underlying mental model dynamics. Ranches that had invested in the company were well respected in their own right as beef producers and individual operators respected each other for their expertise and willingness to invest in the partnership. Until becoming interconnected with the

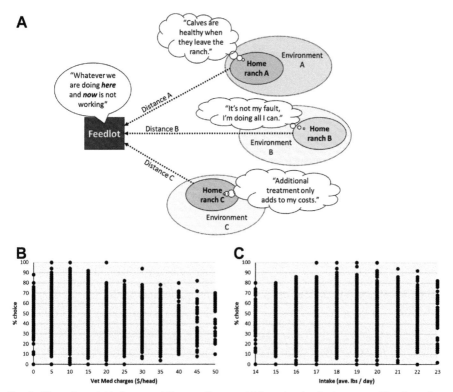

Fig. 9. Mental model inferences (*A*) regarding morbidity crises in the integrated beef production operation, which failed to account for home ranch diversity and geography and contributed to extremely different calf responses to medical treatment (*B*) or average daily intake (*C*).

feedlot as a result of forming the company, home ranches were not accustomed to receiving such negative feedback from the finishing stage of production. Their initial belief was that "we're doing all that we can... certainly the feedlot is the source of the problem." As just described, the subsequent action was to select feedlot data that conformed to their expectation and therefore craft feedlot-centered interventions. Without considering home ranch influence on calf feedlot performance, cow-calf management practices remained business-as-usual. These actions resulted in continued confidence of calves before shipping and continued erosion in feedlot performance, thereby reinforcing the original belief (**Fig. 10**).

The Role of Mental Models as Leverage Points

According to Meadows,[30] improving or changing mental models is one of the highest leverage interventions we can exert on the systems we manage and live in; therefore, it is apt to close this article thinking about interventions to our 2 case studies and possible shifts in mental models about beef production health management. Because 1 case has been successfully resolved, we close with it first.

As described above, the consultant team evaluating the morbidity crisis for the integrated beef production operation, having studied the data and completing their analysis, recommended that the company require preconditioning all calves at the cow-calf ranch-level before shipment to the feedlot and that any morbidity treatment

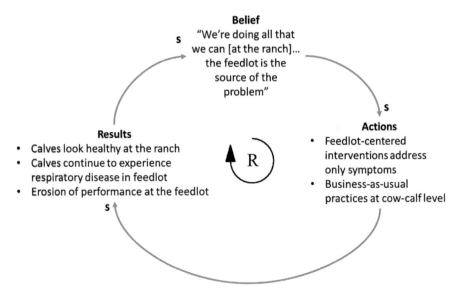

Fig. 10. Belief-action-result loop observed in the integrated beef production morbidity crisis case study.

costs occurring at the feedlot be billed to the home ranch of origin, which the company followed. Through requiring preconditioning, the company began putting all calves on a more even playing field, as calves became better prepared for shipment and performance in the feedlot and therefore more likely to receive a premium price (the "carrot"). By assigning treatment costs to home ranches, operators knew they could not afford to run a subpar preconditioning unit lest they take the financial hit later (the "stick").

When thinking about the industry-wide morbidity crisis, more tact will be needed given the number and variety of stakeholders involved, their roles in the system (and their perceptions of them), and the wider array of external forces that converge at the industry level that make anticipation of and mitigation for unintended consequences much more challenging. Some have proposed greater adoption of backgrounding, preconditioning, or other preparatory methods at the cow-calf or stocker level[8] (similar to the case described previously); better animal husbandry; improved diagnosis for more rapid and individualized treatments; preshipment metaphylaxis (when possible); among other strategies.[8,26] Some of these are constrained biologically. Owing to age and immunologic maturity, yearlings are less likely to receive metaphylactic treatment, and many visual or objective measures of morbidity are unreliable indicators of morbidity diagnoses, which tends to be very inaccurate. Nevertheless, there are some plausible leverage points grounded in mental models worth exploring.

The beef cattle industry as a whole has taken a "data-driven" rather than a "goal-driven" approach. Garrick and Golden[19] state:

"The foundation principles for establishing a sound breeding program, including the prediction of animal performance for economically relevant traits and their incorporation into a single index of aggregate economic merit, have been well established over the last half century. Rather than this goal-based approach, the industry adopted a data-driven approach to the production of genetic

evaluations that has been characterized by an overemphasis on the evaluation of productive traits…with inadequate regard for other economically important traits, such as reproduction, animal health, and feed requirements.

The investigators go on to conclude that current use of genetic-based evaluations has stopped short of any index-based criteria as a basis for animal selection; this is likely due to the plethora of economic incentives (eg, price and premium mechanisms) that reward volume and production quality. One exception is the cow-calf sector, which has developed an indexed criterion for selection of an economically important trait, stayability, an index of the probability of a bull's daughter to successfully join the mature cow herd and remain productive at least until 6 years of age. Not in wide use because of the additional data collection and monitoring requirements over the cow's productive life (currently in use by the Red Angus Association of America. The American Hereford Association uses a similar index, sustained cow fertility, calculated as a cow's ability to stay in the herd producing calves through 12 years), it does show that there is adequate infrastructure and support capacity needed to facilitate wider adoption. Translating the concept of stayability to the terminal calf production line, what if data across key performance traits already in use (such as carcass weight, marbling, and days to finish) could be aggregated with health treatment data to create an index of *finishability*, or the ability of the calf to finish at a certain yield and quality, within a certain amount of time or expected treatment level? Less data would be required relative to stayabilty because the cattle are terminal and most if not all the data exist. Such an addition would not upset current breeding and data collection efforts because it does not seek to overturn existing EPD information structures, but it would allow for new avenues of value creation (eg, premiums based on yield plus "finishabilty" to increase the number of potentially qualified animals to meet retail branded beef offerings aimed at health conscious consumer demands around antibiotic use) with the positive externality of reduced risks of morbidity.

CONCLUSIONS: LESSONS FROM COMPLEX SYSTEMS

Upon reflecting on the beef production health challenges outlined in this article, there are several key principles or characteristics that emerge that are common to all complex systems:

- Cause and effect are distant in time and space and that we often default to blaming others or those outside the system as the cause of the problem rather than examine how we ourselves are causing it[21] (as seen in the integrated beef organization).
- Delays in feedback tend to worsen our ability to intuit behaviors and manage problems,[21,31] worsening our performance over time (as seen in the industry-wide case, where identification of sick animals is already problematic and metaphylactic treatment masks this even further).
- When striving for sustainable interventions, one should admire the problem first before jumping to the immediate and obvious (and often wrong) solutions (ie, "delay your intuitions" until you've surveyed the data you're not even aware of yet[25]).

In this article, we have oriented ourselves to the systems thinking approach, which is grounded in feedback processes and appreciation for the powerful role that mental models exert on how we behave and systems perform. We have highlighted how the systems thinking process may be used to examine contemporary agricultural or natural resource issues—in this case, morbidity in the beef supply chain. Management of such problems is only going to become more complex and challenging due to the array of interconnected ecologic, economic, and social drivers that constitute our systems. Approaches such as these will be needed even more, not less. To continue your journey as a systems thinker, be encouraged that you are not alone. Engage with others who are open-minded and interested in speaking the language of systems. Dig deeper into the mental models that are at work around you. Experiment with the archetypes yourself. Attend a workshop, join a peer group, or find a host of resources online. The systems thinking road may be the one less traveled by, but there are plenty of signposts to guide the way.

CONFLICTS OF INTEREST

The author has nothing to disclose.

ACKNOWLEDGMENTS

Special thanks and appreciation are due to the organizers of this text for the courage to pursue systems thinking as a means to improve scientific and management thought and skill and I am extremely appreciative of their invitation to contribute to such effort. This work was partially supported by USDA's Higher Education Challenge Grant No. 2018-70003-27664 "Curriculum Development for Wicked Problem Solving" and USDA's Research and Extension Experiences for Undergraduates Grant No. 2020-67037-30652 "Research and extension experience in Energy and the Environment across Agricultural Disciplines".

REFERENCES

1. Payne, CA. Fundamentals of Systems Thinking, Veterinary Clinics of North America: Food Animal Practice Volume 38, Number 2, July 2022
2. Smith RA. Impact of disease on feedlot performance: a review. J Anim Sci 1998;76(1):272–4.
3. Wittum TE, Woollen NE, Perino LJ, et al. Relationships among treatment for respiratory tract disease, pulmonary lesions evident at slaughter, and rate of weight gain in feedlot cattle. J Am Vet Med Assoc 1996;209(4):814–8.
4. Larson RL. Effect of cattle disease on carcass traits. J Anim Sci 2005;83(Suppl 13):E37–43.
5. Maday J. "The feedlot death loss conundrum". Drovers CattleNetwork; 2016. Available at: Agweb.com/article/the-feedlot-death-loss-conundrum-NAA-drovers-cattlenetwork.
6. Cooper, D., "Feedyard data reveals higher death losses", Progressive Cattleman, December 24, 2015. Available at: progressivecattle.com/topics/herd-health/feedyard-data-reveals-higher-death-losses.
7. Snowder GD, Van Vleck LD, Cundiff LV, et al. Bovine respiratory disease in feedlot cattle: environmental, genetic, and economic factors. J Anim Sci 2006;84:1999–2008.
8. Nickell JS, White BJ. Metaphylactic antimicrobial therapy for bovine respiratory disease in stocker and feedlot cattle. Vet Clin Food Anim 2010;26:285–301.
9. Vogel GJ, Bokenkroger CD, Rutten-Ramos SC, et al. A retrospective evaluation of animal mortality in US feedlots: rate, timing, and cause of death. Bov Pract 2015;49:113–23.
10. Peel DS. The effect of market forces on bovine respiratory disease. Vet Clin Food Anim 2020;36:497–508.

11. Theurer ME, Johnson MD, Fox T, et al. Bovine respiratory disease during the mid-portion of the feeding period: observations of frequency, timing, and population from the field. Appl Anim Sci 2020;37:52–8.
12. Miles DG. Overview of the North American beef cattle industry and the incidence of bovine respiratory disease (BRD). Anim Health Res Rev 2009;10(2):101–3.
13. Kansas State University. Focus on Feedlots 2021. Department of Animal Sciences and Industry website. Focus on Feedlots monthly reports, KSU. Available at: https://www.asi.k-state.edu/about/newsletters/focuss-on-feedlots/. Accessed November 23, 2021.
14. USDA APHIS Veterinary Services. National Animal Health Monitoring System (NAHMS), Health Management on U.S. Feedlots. 2011. Available at: https://www.aphis.usda.gov/aphis/ourfocus/animalhealth/monitoring-and-surveillance/nahms/NAHMS_Feedlot_Studies. Accessed November 23, 2021.
15. Speer N. What's your cost to keep a cow? 2016. Livestock Marketing Information Center, Lakewood (CO). Available at: https://www.beefmagazine.com/cow-calf/what-s-your-cost-keep-cow. Accessed November 23, 2021.
16. USDA National Agricultural Statistics Service (NASS) - Quick Stats. Available at: https://quickstats.nass.usda.gov/. Accessed November 29, 2021.
17. National Beef Quality Audit, 2011. Available at: https://www.bqa.org/resources/national-beef-quality-audits/past-audits/steer-heifer/2011-national-beef-quality-audit. Accessed November 29, 2021.
18. Speer N. Industry At A Glance: Carcasses grading Prime and Choice hit a record-high. 2015, BEEF Magazine. 2015. Available at: https://www.beefmagazine.com/beef-quality/industry-glance-carcasses-grading-prime-choice-hit-record-high. Accessed November 30, 2021.
19. Garrick DJ, Golden BL. Producing and using genetic evaluations in the Unites States beef industry today. J Anim Sci 2009;87:E11–8.
20. USDA. Beef 2007-2008 Part IV: reference of beef cow-calf management practices in the United States, 2007-08. Riverdale, MD: USDA-APHIS-VS-CEAH-NAHMS; 2010. Available at: https://www.aphis.usda.gov/animal_health/nahms/beefcowcalf/downloads/beef0708/Beef0708_dr_PartIV_1.pdf.
21. Senge PM, Kleiner A, Roberts C, et al. The fifth discipline fieldbook: strategies and tools for building a learning organization. New York: Doubleday; 1994.
22. Kim DH. Systems Archetypes I: diagnosing systemic issues and designing high-leverage interventions. Pegasus Communications, Inc. Available at: https://thesystemsthinker.com/systems-archetypes-i-diagnosing-systemic-issues-and-designing-interventions/.
23. Turner BL, Menendez HM, Gates R, et al. System dynamics modeling for agricultural and natural resource management issues: Review of some past cases and forecasting future roles. Resources 2016;5(4):40.
24. Doyle JK, Ford DN. Mental model concepts for system dynamics research. Syst Dyn Rev 1998;14(1):3–29.
25. Kahneman D. Thinking, fast and slow. New York: Farrar, Straus and Giroux; 2011.
26. Edwards TA. Control methods for bovine respiratory disease for feedlot cattle. Vet Clin Food Anim 2010;26:273–84.
27. Edwards TA. Respiratory diseases of feedlot cattle in the central USA. Bov Pract 1996;30:5–7.
28. Word AB, Wickersham TA, Trubenbach LA, et al. Effects of metaphylaxis on production responses and total antimicrobial use in high-risk beef calves. Appl Anim Sci 2020;36:265–70.

29. Schneider MJ, Tait RG, Busby WB, et al. An evaluation of bovine respiratory disease complex in feedlot cattle: impact on performance and carcass traits using treatment records and lung lesion scores. J Anim Sci 2009;87:1821–7.
30. Meadows DH. Leverage points-places to intervene in a system. In: Thinking in systems: a primer. White River Junction: Chelsea Publishing Company; 2008. p. 145–65.
31. Turner BL, Goodman M, Machen R, et al. Results of beer game trials played by natural resource managers versus students: Does age influence ordering decisions? Systems 2020;8(4):37.

Systems Thinking Perspectives on Stewardship and Our Future

Gerald L. Stokka, DVM, MS[a],*, T. Robin Falkner, DVM[b,c]

KEYWORDS

- Stewardship • Husbandry • Systems thinking • Sustainable

KEY POINTS

- Understanding a stewardship philosophy.
- Applying a systems thinking approach to the use of livestock, land, and people.
- Applying the veterinary oath to the Stewardship practice of veterinary medicine.

STEWARDSHIP

Stewardship is a term that denotes a way of life or alternatively, an ethos of behavior.[1] According to the Merriam-Webster dictionary, stewardship is defined as "the careful and responsible management of things entrusted to one's care," whereas the definition of ethos can be stated as "the distinguishing character, sentiment, moral nature, or guiding beliefs of a person, group, or institution." The usage of these terms is found in different contexts, such as environmental stewardship, or a company sharing its business ethos, which often accompany and are expressed in marketing campaigns. Agriculture can be defined as the science or practice of farming/ranching, including husbandry of the soil for the growing of crops and the rearing of animals to provide food and a host of other goods. The use of the terms stewardship and ethos, when applied in this context, implies the use of land, people, and livestock in such a manner that the goods produced will be the output of a system in which long-term sustainability is enhanced, such that the next generation of caretakers are the beneficiaries of the stewardship of previous generations.

The systems thinking discipline is a set of synergistic investigative skills, used to improve the capability of identifying and understanding complex adaptive systems,

[a] Department of Animal Science, College of Agriculture, Food Systems and Natural Resources, North Dakota State University, 207C Morrill Hall, NDSU Department 7630, PO Box 6050, Fargo, ND 58108-6050, USA; [b] CattleFlow Consulting, Christiana, TN, USA; [c] Elanco Animal Health, Greenfield, IN, USA
* Corresponding author.
E-mail address: gerald.stokka@ndsu.edu

Vet Clin Food Anim 38 (2022) 201–207
https://doi.org/10.1016/j.cvfa.2022.02.002
0749-0720/22/© 2022 Elsevier Inc. All rights reserved.

predicting their behaviors, and devising modifications to them to produce desired changes. These skills work together as a system.[2]

How does the philosophy of stewardship and the perspective of systems thinking blend together?

The 2 concepts become interconnected as the ethos of the entire system with all its parts within its boundaries, providing policy makers with guidance to implement careful, moral, and responsible management. Ultimately, application of stewardship requires that resources entrusted to agriculturalists within a system must be used in a manner that not only permits future generations to have similar opportunities but also assures it; this implies that unless the system operates with stewardship principles as part of its ethos, it is destined to be unsustainable.

HOW SYSTEMS STEWARDSHIP IMPACTS THE USE OF LAND AND LIVESTOCK

The guiding ethos of agricultural stewardship principles that follow certainly overlap and provide foundations for the logic and behavior relating to good stewardship.

1. Ownership: Livestock and wildlife are sentient beings, with wildlife considered public usage, whereas private ownership of livestock is proffered. In cultures that recognize private property rights deeded land is privately owned and will be sold/transferred to subsequent generations. Both privately and publicly owned resources are to be managed with care and wisdom, knowing that land is irreplaceable, and livestock are an important part of a complex adaptive system that benefits society. Their use provides humanity with a system-friendly, renewable food source and a multitude of valuable by-products.
2. Responsibility: A steward accepts responsibility for the care of livestock and the preservation of the land and its uses. Accepting responsibility is a characteristic of leadership and provides direct access to accountability.
3. Accountability: Good stewards are accountable regarding the use of resources entrusted to them. To give an account for how the system has been managed implies transparency and a willingness to teach others.
4. Reward: Whatever you do, work at it with all your heart, knowing that you may provide opportunities for following generations. Good stewards are often sought out to be involved with many other endeavors. Others will notice good stewardship behavior and learn from it.[3]

The intentional application of these principles leads to good stewardship. Owners have limited rights; stewards have responsibilities. The Torah refers to human authority over the animals, using the term "dominion."[4] The term dominion does not imply domination, but carries with it responsibility and accountability. Responsibility as part of good animal stewardship is managing available resources such that:

- Livestock are provided the nutritional needs to meet the animal requirements regarding thirst, hunger, and malnutrition, and have access to water and a diet sufficient to maintain health and vigor.
- During times of stress such as parturition, weaning, handling, transportation, and commingling, it is critical to provide sufficient management and husbandry expertise to support animal well-being.
- Disease and injury are minimal and promptly treated, and the risk of such is minimized.[5] Accountability is essential for the agricultural steward. However, the potential for the reward of good stewardship is the motivation and lifeblood of the caretaker lifestyle. A good steward takes pride in the work related to land and livestock management. Anything less than this creates greater separation and

potential mistrust between the steward, the public consumer, and those that question the resource use of ranching. Good stewardship must be the standard, and evidence of lower standards must be identified, unlearned, and changed.

HOW OUR WORLDVIEW IMPACTS STEWARDSHIP

Numerous uses and reasons for the keeping of animals have existed over time including, but are not limited to, food sources, transportation, various forms of work, and religious customs. However, the primary output of animals in modern agricultural systems is food for human consumption. In developed countries the system must meet the high standards for nutrition and safety, such as approved nutritional composition labels, food safety assurance, environmental impact, animal well-being, and land use. In countries in which the system of food production tends toward subsistence levels, the standards may be less uniform, but nutrition and food safety are still of importance.

The guiding cultural use of animals is found not only in Western cultures but also in others. In societies adhering to Judeo-Christian principles, the biblical approval of animal use for food is found.

In Mongolian culture the use of animals is similar because animals are used for food, fiber, and labor. A livestock festival occurs every year in the spring, to celebrate the prosperity enjoyed as a result of livestock. The Greeks domesticated goats, dogs, horses, pigs, and sheep. Large horses first appeared in Greek times. Greeks developed the first horseshoes in AD fourth century, and sheep were raised for their fine wool. Chickens were raised in Egypt and China for meat and eggs by 1400 BCE, Greeks used them as a source of food, and they were already established in Britain by the time the Romans arrived (43 CE). Subsequently, they were brought to the New World by explorers and conquistadors.[6]

The choice to remove animal food products and protein from diets is known as vegetarianism. In antiquity, human populations only relied on strictly vegetarian diets because of poverty or scarcity of food animals. More recently, vegetarianism in all its forms seems enveloped in philosophy related to animal rights, religion, hygiene, environment, and even a desire for racial purity. There are many different degrees of vegetarianism. Vegans avoid everything animal—clothing, lacto (allows dairy), ovo (allows eggs), pollo (allows poultry), and pesco (allows fish). Also included in this mix are those that consume all animal protein but exclude what is considered red meat.[6]

It is clear from a biological standpoint that humans have the capability to use both plants and foods of animal origin in diets. Food derived from animals is very nutrient dense, because calories and protein contained in small measure of weight is much higher than that in any plant food.[7] Animals that convert humanly indigestible plants into a palatable human food are highly valued. Food animals that perform this conversion are a critical component of a system that is environment friendly and leads to more efficient use of nonarable land.

HOW STEWARDSHIP IMPACTS OUR RELATIONSHIPS WITH PEOPLE, LIVESTOCK, AND FOOD
System Approach

There are people inhabiting every continent with the exception of Antarctica. Food preferences are very diverse depending on the climate, geography, philosophy, and culture. In developed societies, food is shipped some distances to meet food preferences. In large cities and urban areas transportation of food is a necessity; however, it allows for a great menu of personal food choices to meet nutritional needs. Less-developed societies produce and consume most of the food locally, because infrastructure is inadequate for efficient transportation of imported goods. In these less developed societies, personal food choices are restricted and nutritional needs may be unmet. Societies with a stewardship philosophy regarding the use of land and livestock view food production from a holistic or systems approach. This approach quantifies what nature has provided, and places limits on inputs such that production is optimized rather than maximized. Policies developed without regard to reality of food production will result in a decrease in food availability and concomitant increased costs.[8,9]

Stewardship of the Veterinary Profession

"Being admitted to the profession of veterinary medicine I solemnly swear to use my scientific knowledge and skills for the benefit of society, through the protection of animal health and welfare, the prevention and relief of animal suffering, the conservation of animal resources, the promotion of public health and the advancement of medical knowledge."

"I will practice my profession conscientiously, with dignity, and in keeping with the principles of veterinary medical ethics. I accept as a lifelong obligation the continual improvement of my professional knowledge and competence."[10]

It is clear from the veterinary oath that the ethos of the veterinary profession is also defined in stewardship terms. To benefit society bridges the gap with the public and promotes stewardship of animals by addressing animal health, animal welfare, and the prevention and relief of animal suffering. The conservation of animal resources addresses the stewardship use of land, water and people, and the statement regarding public health addresses the responsibility of the steward to those not involved in the production of goods.

The livestock veterinary practitioner who has dedicated all or part of the business to the management and health of livestock understands the business tension that exists when production management decisions are complicated by the requirements of a for-profit business and the well-being of animals. An example is the procurement of feeder calves perceived to be at a high risk of developing respiratory disease. The tension is between purchase price, which is lower due to the perceived risk of disease, the availability of animals at that price, and the expectation of significant morbidity, mortality, and chronic illness in this group of animals. As a business, the purchase price offered will be influenced by the number of animals predicted to become ill, and require treatment, along with loss of performance, and by the number of animals predicted to die or become chronically ill versus those that remain healthy. To the veterinary practitioner the recognition of the business model and the challenge and opportunity to provide a positive influence may result in conflict with the business. How does the ethos of the veterinary oath align with accepting a predicted illness, death loss, and the use of therapeutic products as long as a financial profit can be realized? The stewardship conflict for the veterinary practitioner is one of providing advice to management, which reduces the risk of illness and death loss not to exceed a certain target, but not addressing the stewardship responsibility regarding antibiotic use, and welfare of livestock to reduce their stress and suffering.

Difficult issues often present opportunities for change. The aforementioned example presents an opportunity to manage the system rather than each piece independently. Systems thinking veterinarians recognize that clinical disease is usually the result of disruptions in the system resulting from a series of risk factors that overwhelm normal defense mechanisms designed to protect the animal. The etiologic agent may be important to identify; however, it may only be symptomatic of perturbation in the system. Stressors in the system must be identified and managed. Stress occurs from front to back, beginning with and during the original production premises. In addition, stressors occur during the procurement system, the transportation, the arrival environment, the arrival nutrition, the pen size, animal density, and the ability of the operation to contain high-risk animals with enough space and limited numbers to reduce the psychological stress associated with resocializing animals by group.[11,12]

In pathogen stress work done by Hodgson and colleagues, bovine respiratory disease (BRD) in unvaccinated cattle was reproduced by bovine herpes virus-1 infection followed 4 days later by aerosol challenge with *Mannheimia haemolytica*. This model induced clinical signs of respiratory disease in unvaccinated calves with a mortality of 30% to 70%.[13] This BRD model along with weaning alone or transport alone versus weaning plus transport resulted in mortality rates 2 times greater than that of weaning or transport alone. Additional stressors significantly altered the viral-bacterial synergy resulting in fatal BRD. Under field conditions vaccination on arrival alone produces disappointing results in reducing the risk of BRD.[14] This is the case especially with the use of vaccines containing bacterial antigens. Evidence suggests the ability of the immune system to respond to vaccines against potential bacterial pathogens that are also part of the normal host flora is limited at best in preventing infection or reducing inflammatory damage to lung tissue. In a systems approach addressing management of vaccine efficacy and product selection or timing of vaccine administration of newly arrived calves is of limited value.[14,15] Livestock systems veterinarians must have the ability to identify and focus on the entire system and offer advice on potential leverage points for reducing the risk of illness by educating and training caretakers to recognize the signs of wellness in calves as well as signs of early illness.[16]

Operations with a business model of managing health in highly commingled, transported groups of calves have a need to recognize the systemic disturbances that result from too many animals arriving at the facility in a short period.[11] Large group size can exacerbate stress disturbances. For example, pathogen stress is enhanced when individual animals are incubating, infected, and shedding organisms to penmates. The greater the number of animals within a confined space the greater the opportunity for transmission and for the infectious pathogen dose to transmit to uninfected yet stressed animals.[12,17] In addition, biocontainment becomes less manageable and caretaker stress is increased due to too many untreated and previously treated animals needing observation and medical intervention. Limiting numbers of calves per pen or groups per pen may reduce the stress level of the entire group. The stress and concomitant signs of illness are more easily recognized and managed in more pens with fewer animals. In addition, paying more attention to the behavior of wellness in animals may result in an increase in the ability to assess illness in animals that actually need therapeutic intervention,[1] particularly in the 2- to 4-week early arrival period. During this period, observing animal behavior indicating wellness can be of great importance. Animals that are well will demonstrate curiosity with pen-mates and humans, will interact with other animals by grooming themselves and others and of course moving to the feed source, eating and drinking. Manage the animals, the disturbance stress in the system regarding facilities, pathogens, nutrition, and the environment, to provide the best opportunity to minimize the risk of stress and optimize wellness.

SUMMARY

Systems/stewardship practicing veterinarians have the opportunity to provide essential services to livestock operations beyond the technical skills and product-driven services that have been the mainstay of veterinary education and practice for the previous 50 years. Our veterinary oath demands more from our profession, and our clients demand more relevance from our unique systems stewardship knowledge and experience.

DISCLOSURE

The authors have nothing to disclose.

REFERENCES

1. Descombes CREH. Before ethics?: A study of the ethos of the medical profession. 2001:6-7. 2002.
2. Stephens EC. Review of systems thinking concepts and their potential value in animal science research. J Anim Sci 2021;99(2):1–7.
3. Cattlemen's stewardship review. Denver, CO: Cattlemen's Beef Board and National Cattlemen's Beef Association; 2017. p. 1–64. Available at: https://www.beefitswhatsfordinner.com/Media/BIWFD/Docs/beef-csr-report-2017-final.pdf. Accessed January 10, 2022.
4. The Torah.: Genesis 1:26. E-artnow; Feb 18, 2021.
5. Farm animal welfare in great britain: past, present and future. London: Farm Animal Welfare Council Area 5A,9 Millbank, c/o Nobel House, 17 Smith Square, SW1P 3JR. 2009. Available at: https://assets.publishing.service.gov.uk/government/uploads/system/uploads/attachment_data/file/319292/Farm_Animal_Welfare_in_Great_Britain_-_Past_Present_and_Future.pdf. Accessed January 10, 2022.
6. Kiple KF, Kriemhild Coneè Ornelas. The cambridge World history of food/the cambridge World history of food. Cambridge University Press; 2000. https://doi.org/10.1017/CHOL9780521402156.
7. Roesel K. Sustainable food systems and agriculture: how animal sourced foods contribute to a healthy diet. In: Encyclopedia of food security and sustainability. Elsevier; 2019. p. 299–309.
8. FAO. Livestock and agroecology how they can support the transition towards sustainable food and agriculture. 2018. Available at: https://www.fao.org/3/I8926EN/i8926en.pdf. Accessed October 8, 2021.
9. Solzhenitsyn, Aleksandr Isaevich. The Gulag Archipelago, 1918–1956 : an experiment in literary investigation / Aleksandr I. Solzhenitsyn ; translated from the Russian by Thomas P. Whitney Harper & Row New York, 1974.
10. Veterinarian's Oath. American veterinary medical association. Available at: https://www.avam.org/resources-tools/avma-policies/veterinarians-oath. Accessed January 11, 2022.
11. Duff GC, Galyean ML. Board-invited review: recent advances in management of highly stressed, newly received feedlot cattle. J Anim Sci 2007;85(3):823–40.
12. Chen Y, Arsenault R, Napper S, et al. Models and methods to investigate acute stress responses in cattle. Animals (Basel) 2015;5(4):1268–95.
13. Hodgson P, Aich P, Manuja A, et al. Effect of stress on viral-bacterial synergy in bovine respiratory disease: novel mechanisms to regulate inflammation. Comp Funct Genomics 2005;6(4):244–50.
14. O'Connor AM, Hu D, Totton SC, et al. A systematic review and network meta-analysis of bacterial and viral vaccines, administered at or near arrival at the feedlot, for control of bovine respiratory disease in beef cattle. Anim Health Res Rev 2019;20(2):143–62.

15. Angelos J, Elizalde P, Griebel P. Bovine immune responses to moraxella bovis and moraxella bovoculi following vaccination and natural or experimental infections. Vet Clin North Am Food Anim Pract 2021;37(2):253–66.
16. Jackson K, Carstens G, Tedeschi L, et al. Changes in feeding behavior patterns and dry matter intake before clinical symptoms associated with bovine respiratory disease in growing bulls. J Anim Sci 2016;94(4):1644–52.
17. Enriquez D, Hötzel MJ, Ungerfeld R. Minimizing the stress of weaning of beef calves: a review. Acta Vet Scand 2011;53(1):28.

Systems Assessment of Beef Sustainability

Jason E. Sawyer, PhD

KEYWORDS

- Sustainable • Systems thinking • Indicators

KEY POINTS

- Sustainability is an estimate of the persistence of a system over time, and its assessment is a forecasting problem.
- Food production systems, like beef production, are disperse and complex, making forecasting difficult.
- Assessment of sustainability can be improved using systems thinking.
- Systems evaluation aids in identification of nonlinearity and delays in system feedbacks, which can improve foresight and forecasting over defined time frames.
- Systems-based analysis frameworks are likely to yield improved indicators of sustainability and avoid the unintended consequences of driving policy and management through inadequate forecasting capability.

INTRODUCTION

Terms related to "sustainability," "sustainable development," and "sustainable systems" have permeated the public discourse. Businesses have seized on them through a sense of corporate responsibility to society; from a strategic marketing perspective; or in reaction to regulatory, customer, or consumer pressure (real, anticipatory, or perceived). Activists in a variety of arenas use these terms to galvanize public action or reaction; and governments and nongovernment organizations have adopted these terms in promulgation of and advocacy for public policy, to the extent that the term has had its meaning diluted.[1]

For individual operators and the beef industry as a whole, the notion of sustainability and the public perception of agriculture have become increasingly contentious. Elements of this tension include the lack of a common, valid, and defensible definition of "sustainability"; the potential for false inference from insufficient indicators; and the difficulties inherent in the assessment of complex systems. The objective of this article is to use systems thinking approaches to address these issues and develop a framework from which assessment and management might proceed.

King Ranch® Institute for Ranch Management, Texas A&M University, Kingsville, 700 University Blvd. MSC 137, Kingsville, TX 78363, USA
E-mail address: jason.sawyer@tamuk.edu

Vet Clin Food Anim 38 (2022) 209–217
https://doi.org/10.1016/j.cvfa.2022.03.002
0749-0720/22/© 2022 Elsevier Inc. All rights reserved.

DEFINITION OF SUSTAINABILITY

"Sustain" is a verb, meaning to provide for existence, continuance; to support persistence. "Sustainable," the adjective form, means possessing the ability to be sustained or persist; sustainability, the noun form of the term, is then the ability itself (ie, the ability to persist or be sustained). Sustainability, therefore, is a property of a system.

Many interpretations of sustainability are associated with the adjective form, "sustainable." The United Nations[2] defined sustainable development as "meeting the needs of the present without compromising the ability of future generations to meet their own needs." This commission indicates that limits are conditions of the present state of technology and "social organization" relative to resource use and allocation. Although this definition has received criticism, it in many ways serves as a basis for many concepts currently associated with sustainability.

One of the earliest uses of this term in its modern context of global systems was in the report "Limits to Growth,"[3] which also strongly attached the term to policy consideration. Drawing from the multifactorial elements described under "sustainable development," the concept of 3 pillars, domains, or dimensions of sustainability emerged, and their representation in a Venn-like diagram was introduced.[4] In the 1990 Farm Bill, the US Congress included these elements in its definition of sustainable agriculture: "...must meet human food and fiber needs, enhance environmental quality and natural resources, maximize efficiency of use of non-renewable resources, sustain economic vitality of agricultural operations, and enhance quality of life for society as a whole." Sustainable agriculture has been alternately defined as "capable of maintaining productivity and usefulness to society indefinitely,"[5] a definition that is more directly drawn from the literal meaning of the term.

As additional properties, conditions, constraints and required outflows are added to define a "sustainable" system, they evolve into philosophic, positional, or value statements rather than descriptions of the properties of a system.[6] This shift loads the discussion of sustainability, as alternate views are perceived as attacks on a value system rather than debate on descriptions of system properties. Finding mechanisms to describe sustainability independently of this transition is vital to the effective incorporation of these concepts into actionable strategies or solutions.

SUSTAINABILITY AND SYSTEMS

Systems are described by their boundaries (what is and is not contained within the system), components, the interactions and feedbacks among their components, and their products or rates of production. These systems are dynamic in time, self-organizing, path-dependent and state-dependent, and adaptive. As a result, the responses of the system to inputs are often nonlinear and counterintuitive, and systems may be resistant to efforts to change their functions.[7] These are "emergent" properties, which are derived from the operation of the system as a whole and may not be directly observable by examining a single component.

The persistence of a system over time, or its continuing capacity to generate its product(s), can be considered an emergent property because it cannot be observed in an instantaneous metric. Rather, sustainability can only be assessed over time; a system that currently exists and functions (eg, generates an output), and has done so for some amount of time from the past until the present, has exhibited sustainability until the present time. Its capacity to continue to do so (maintenance of the property of sustainability) requires a forecast of future events, based on the current system state and relationships among the components of the system. Evaluating the "sustainability" of a system into the future is therefore a forecasting problem,[8] and much of the contention over "sustainability" issues can be framed as challenges associated with forecasting: what measure to forecast (such as output, input utilization), validity of models used to generate the forecasts, timescale(s) of relevance, and uncertainties associated with system boundaries and representation. It is more useful from an operational perspective to consider the *likelihood* that a given system is sustainable, *over a defined timeframe*. Actions that alter the system, or exogenous shocks or nudges to the system, may increase, reduce, or not alter the estimated likelihood of persistence, given uncertainties associated with its assessment.

Systems analysis, from problem solving approaches such as systems thinking to complex modeling of systems dynamics, offers tools to address the question of sustainability because they offer ways to develop foresight of system behavior over time and to evaluate the levels of uncertainty in associated forecasts.

From a systems perspective, sustainability is often viewed in terms of resource constraints. Resource constraints on global output, relative to global population demand, are the "Limits to Growth" (3). The systems archetype of limits to growth,[7] describes a condition in which some required resource or other constraining factor is depleted and results in collapse of the system. Within this framework, "sustainability" might be characterized as the likelihood of remaining within the implied limits. The limits to growth archetype are analogous to the ecological concept of "carrying capacity." Carrying capacity is the level at which consumption is equal to, but does not exceed, resource supply or regeneration[6]; operating the system at that level is likely to be sustainable over reasonable timeframes.

A simplistic view of the limits to growth archetype is that if a resource is consumed, then at some point, it must become exhausted; therefore, the system cannot be sustained. This simplistic view is necessarily nihilistic; no known system is infinitely sustainable. Even the sun, which is the source (ultimately) of most energy and assimilative power on Earth, will eventually burn out and thus render the Earth system unsustainable. This issue can be in part remedied by estimating the likelihood of persistence over more pragmatic timeframes. This view may also fail to consider the wide-ranging nature of the implied limits and resources, the opportunities for substitution and replacement, or the renewability of certain resources. Together, these characteristics may confer "policy resistance" to the system,[7] in which the system adapts to maintain its function. Although the description of this character has a negative connotation, it might also be viewed as resilience, the adaptation of a complex system to persist in the face of shocks.

Systems analysis, by incorporating multiple variables and their interactions, can also accommodate broader interpretations of sustainability by expanding system boundaries.[9] The commonly used tripartite notion of sustainability being composed of environmental, economic, and social dimensions is well accommodated in a systems framework, where these elements subsystems that interact. This is an important feature because it avoids the reductive problem of compartmentalization, in which maximization of one component may be detrimental to the larger system. It also helps to illustrate the nature of delays and operating timescales in the system because each of these subsystems may have differing delays or reaction times. These subsystems are common to many reporting methodologies, including triple bottom line accountancy,[10] and all arise from a common philosophic base around sustainability issues.[10]

The economic subsystem describes the mechanism for allocation of resources, without which outflows will cease or consumption will accelerate. At finer scales, failure to adequately cover the costs of outflows will cause the system to falter or limit output. At a large scale, economic considerations might be considered systemic regulators, affecting the allocation of resources to systems of higher implicit value.

The social dimension incorporates philosophic and ethical considerations regarding societal expectations and interactions. In some cases, elements considered under the social dimension might predict the sustainability of human resources; in others, they might consider the reality that "societal acceptance" of system elements may be necessary conditions of continuance, and thus persistence of the system. Measures often associated with the social dimension may the most challenging to validate empirically.

Clearly, elements of these dimensions may be related; resource consumption and resulting scarcity escalate costs; increasing costs of system outputs may jeopardize quality of life for vulnerable populations; other populations may or may not accept the methods or mechanisms of production and resource utilization, thus reducing demand and capacity to service production costs. Interrelated measures or methods of accounting for interdimensional relationships in sustainability assessment improve the capacity to forecast persistence.

Boundary considerations include the consideration of externalities. If an outflow of the system (waste, pollution) threatens the resources that sustain the system, then this implies a limit to growth or a collapse unless the situation is remedied; this is internal to the system so long as the stocks and use of the resource are considered. A feedback loop in the structure relates the level of the resource to its consumption, and this may result in impacts on the physical function of the system (direct output) or the economic subsystem (rationing of supply through price; increased costs, reduced consumption).

Alternately, the outflow may not have direct impact on the functioning of the system, but affects some other external but parallel system negatively, and compromise the external system likelihood of persistence. In this case, the system boundary can be expanded to include the parallel system, but this may add unnecessary complexity. However, this externality does affect the societal perspective of the relative value of the products of the 2 systems, and thus including social license can serve as a proxy for the impact of externalities.[11] If society values the persistence of the alternate system more than the primary system, it may demand the cessation of the primary system—antisustainability. Inclusion of the social dimension within the boundaries of the primary system is an acknowledgment of this linkage and internalizes these effects. The variance in societal value judgment makes this element difficult to forecast, and society's capacity to rationally evaluate the material relationship between the 2 systems becomes a substantial threat to persistence. The unintended consequences of this are important when the primary system is a food production system, itself material to the persistence of the population.

INDICATORS OF SUSTAINABILITY

If "sustainability" of a given system is a desired property, measurements that are effective predictors of persistence are needed if the system is to be managed.[12] Although significant effort has been applied to the development indicators for "sustainability" and "sustainable development" during the last 50 years, few of these have been effectively operationalized across the beef industry, and even fewer have been critically evaluated. In many cases, assessments (eg, energy yield, carbon footprint, water footprint, and so forth) that have been used to describe other systems have been deployed[6,13,14] effectively. However, these methodologies may be impractical for enterprise-level use on a broad scale. Empirically valid proxies are perhaps more desirable and more feasible in management systems. Gross resource consumption (or waste emissions) is often used as a sustainability indicator, and measures of this type are considered "core" indicators in sustainability reporting by the Global

Reporting Initiative[15]; however, in the absence of a scaling variable (ie, consumption relative total resource in existence) or other relevant comparator, these measures are not meaningful predictors in isolation. Ratios, time series measures, or other means are required to place gross measures into context and make them applicable for management.[16]

Predictors, performance indicators, are only relevant if they are indeed predictive. Dale and colleagues[17] suggest a list of criteria that may serve as an effective guide in selecting indicators of sustainability, and Costanza and Patten[8] suggest framing the question of developing indicators around 3 key questions:

1. What system, characteristic of the system, or outflow from the system should persist?
2. How long should the system persist?
3. When can the system be assessed to determine whether or not it has persisted?

The first may be the most straightforward. Answering this question defines a set of objectives for assessment. Because most large systems consist of nested or hierarchical subsystems, the same set of questions can be applied to subsystems to develop additional indicators relevant to the subsystem. However, because the higher order system may be robust to change (ie, the failure of one subsystem does not necessarily cause the demise of the larger system[7]), care should be taken to define relationships that can be quantified or empirically demonstrated. It is important to note that many "indicators" that are often cited in reference to sustainability do not consider the output of the system. This can lead to a call to "abolish the system" because it is consumptive or perceived to threaten human sustainability, failing to acknowledge that the outflow of the system may be itself a necessary element of population sustainability.

The question of time dimension may be more challenging. As with any forecast, near-term predictions are likely to be more accurate than long-term predictions. No known system can last infinitely, but it is impossible to define a desired time limitation on the human population. Thus, although "forever" may be the implication of sustainability, consideration of this question may also help to place a more realistic context on assessment. To resolve these conflicts, indicators that can be assessed routinely, at both short, intermediate, and long-term time scales, can be used to define trends in the subsystems (shorter time scales) and metasystems (longer time scales) of food production. Alternately, the sensitivity of the indicator to trajectories in related variables can be used to project system response to shocks or to estimate trends in time. It is imperative that such analyses are repeated frequently, as new information, technical solutions, or relationships among variables may greatly alter the forecasts. The inclusion of systems dynamics and related considerations can improve foresight, the understanding of factors that can affect the future state of the system, and therefore refine forecasting.

Finally, because the actual "sustainability" of a system can only be evaluated post hoc, some determination of future assessment points is valuable so that trajectory can be evaluated, and the suitability of indicators validated.

CONCEPTS APPLIED TO AGRICULTURE

If the primary role of agriculture is to provide food and fiber to support the human population, then the outflow of food from the system can be defined as the outflow to be sustained; alternately, the ability to supply food sufficient to meet the needs of the population might be the characteristic of the system to be sustained. If the system and its components cannot fulfill this need, they are not viable and change is required (a feedback loop exists). This important notion—adaptation or system evolution to sustain the desired outflow—is related to the need to consider output in sustainability assessment.[8]

Individuals have a base food requirement; thus, a minimum threshold of food production per capita can be established to meet this requirement, or to achieve a target level of surfeit above it assumed to confer "quality of life" rather than survival. Because a minimum below which the population cannot be sustained exists, the indicator (food per capita) has a directional relation; reducing food production per capita is negative to the likelihood of sustaining the population, increasing it is positive to the likelihood of sustaining the population. An appropriate time scale for forecasting this indicator might be related to the time scale over which population dynamics can be reliably forecast.

Food production per capita can be increased in 2 ways: increasing food output or reducing population. Population reduction through overt action as a mechanism to increase sustainability violates a fundamental premise of the system (sustaining or supporting the population). However, population stabilization (or even reduction) that results from other systemic factors such as voluntarily reduced birth rates (as observed in many industrialized nations) should be considered in forecasts.

Particular production systems and the associated strategies, tactics, and technologies applied within these systems can be described in terms of resource utilization and product outflow. Applying economic values to the set of inputs and outflows allows description of the system in economic terms, and the joint description of the biological and economic features of the system is necessary to assess sustainability. Thus, ratios of output to resource utilization, and the associated costs or values per unit, may serve to integrate the components of the system (resources) with the feature of the system (output) for which sustainability is desired.[16]

Resource utilization can be measured in several ways. Resources of public concern might include fossil fuel consumption, nonrenewable water consumption, land (especially arable land) utilization, or consumption of other resources of concern. Resource utilization indicators should be developed as ratios; quantity of resources consumed per unit of output (resource use intensity), or units of output per units of resources consumed (resource efficiency). These indicators may be especially useful in comparing management alternatives or predicting the outcomes of management changes such as intensification. Many firms may have data required to develop these indicators in hand or could easily append current systems to include its collection.

Economic indicators within the system can be described as cost functions. Because costs represent resource consumption, similar ratios can be applied. In most cases, cost ratios with units of production should respond directly with resource ratios, that is, cost efficiency and resource use efficiency are correlated. Deviations from this relationship are likely to be temporal and reflect volatility in resource pricing, and thus simultaneous estimation of both indicators is likely to confer some additional element of anticipatory value to impending system changes or allow the forecasting of the response of the system to various shocks. Additionally, price data per unit can be compared with cost data as an indicator of the firm's economic sustainability. Most firms already track this indicator.

Social sustainability indicators should also include the object function (food per capita) as a priority indicator. This is often ignored in current sustainability measures. Although it is intuitive that gross output or production per capita is a meaningful metric as the sector or industry level, it is not meaningful at the firm level. However, if a baseline per capita target is established, then output from a firm can be characterized in "food units" or similar measure as a scaling variable. As with other dimensions, ratios might be more meaningful, such as the amount of product per unit of resource input or the accumulated cost of a unit of output. Baber and colleagues[18] describe the Net Protein Contribution of beef production systems, and this indicator can be estimated at the firm level. Such indicators scale output to resource use and illustrate the social benefit of the system.

Measures of social acceptability may be difficult to generate at the firm level; proxy values can likely be generated from sector or industry level data if demand information and the estimation of demand elasticity for specific product lines can be collected. As products with attributes that differ primarily in terms of perceived social acceptability are marketed, market size and demand functions are illustrative of true social accept-ability—these functions measure how persons behave, not how they claim they will behave. Thus, as firms consider management changes, they may be able to forecast the likely effects of selecting alternate strategies on this dimension of sustainability by comparing systems adjusted for product demand functions.

An additional element relevant to social sustainability revolves around animal well-being. Indicators in this area should be constructed so that they can be expressed relative to the output function and should meet the criterion of unambiguous evaluation. Examples might include measures already commonly tracked, such as morbidity and mortality rates, and their trends over time. Expressing these per unit of beef produced rather than per head or in aggregate might provide more context and comparability across systems. Benchmarking across other systems might also prove valuable in this dimension. For example, although morbidity rate might be perceived as an indicator that cattle were in poor health, comparing morbidity rate within a system to the illness rate or proportion of employees in the United States that took at least one "sick" day off from work might create more context. In 2004, 46.6% of United States workers aged between 19 and 64 years had to miss at least 1 day of work due to illness. If those reporting illness, but not sick days, are included, the total is increased to 69.6%.[19] This is analogous to morbidity rate and might suggest that morbidity rates in production systems are relatively low, or that the "well-being" of American workers is relatively lower than that of American cattle.

Heitschmidt and colleagues[6] calculated energy ratios (food energy yield per "cultural" energy input) for beef production systems. In this report, cultural energy is a measure of direct and indirect fossil fuel utilization because it considers the energy inputs in fuel, fertilizers, machinery, and so forth across both feed and cattle production systems. These authors evaluated systems of increasing intensity within 3 production strategies. Intensity of production in this study was reflected by increasing days in a feedyard within a given operating strategy. Because increasing days on feed increased purchased feed usage and machinery and fuel inputs, it reflects an increase in total energy inputs into the production system as intensity is increased. However, in all cases, energy yield increased by 50% to 60% when comparing the lowest to highest intensity systems. Thus, although more total energy was consumed, the marginal energy yield was sufficient to offset inputs and resulted in more energy efficient production. Intensification improved this indicator of sustainability, reducing fuel usage per food unit. In terms of sustainability of a system, increasing the efficiency of utilization of finite resources is a goal of sustainable production according to USDA.[5] It is also notable that resource utilization is a proxy for cost when considered at concurrent time points or on real rather than nominal dollars. Higher energy yield thus translates to lower production costs per unit of output, although total costs per animal might be greater. This is a social benefit as a greater proportion of consumers have access to the product at a lower cost.

The methodology of the referenced study[6] did not use a complete life cycle analysis. However, the energy yields estimated are analogous (adjusting for different units of measure across studies) to those reported by Capper[13] or Rotz and colleagues[14] for comparable systems. Empirical data must be used to develop the relationships and models required for life cycle analysis (LCA); cross validation of LCA studies affirms the validity of the models, and the elements of the model inputs can thus be extracted as proxy indicators by managers.

When comparing beef productions systems across time, productivity increases (output per animal) were linked to reductions in greenhouse gas emission and carbon footprint.[13,20] Emissions (and thus footprinting) metrics are difficult to obtain in real time by individual firms; therefore, directly observable measures that provide reasonable approximation are desirable. Energy use intensity (the inverse of energy efficiency) is a direct proxy for greenhouse gas emissions and carbon footprint per unit of outflow. Because increases in intensity are expected to increase outputs, one can predict the response to intensity impacts on sustainability indicators by estimating the change in output due to intensification, and by estimating the increase in resources required to implement the management change. Because these values are relatively straightforward to estimate, a realistic indication of sustainability impacts of an intensification step can be determined. As each of these resources has cost, an estimate of the impact of intensification on indicators of economic sustainability is straightforward to estimate. In fact, this approach to analysis of alternatives is commonplace.

Most examples in the literature support the concept that increasing intensity increases resources use efficiency, although these same steps typically increase total resource or energy consumption because output from the system is also increased. This applies to all resources considered, from land and water to fossil fuels. Intensification in management reduced land use for dairy production by 90% and the number of cows required to produce a constant milk supply by 79%,[20] leading to 63% reductions in carbon footprint. Arguably, much of the research and development of modern agricultural systems has been aimed at reducing the resource utilization required to produce a unit of food, a central indicator of sustainability. We have simply referred to this objective by a different name—production efficiency. Using the tools of systems dynamics is likely to enable an expansion of system boundaries, helping to gain foresight about how improvements in resource use may simply delay, rather than avoid systemic failure, and to more clearly illuminate tradeoffs and offer foresight that allows the design of systems with increasing likelihood of persistence.

SUMMARY

A systems analysis framework is essential for the assessment of sustainability of food production, and this analysis framework offers a method to derive effective predictors of persistence as valid metrics of sustainability. Unfortunately, the tendency of the public to evaluate single, gross indicators, failing to account for system complexity, the necessity of system outputs, scaling variables, or time dimensions, can result in the formation of policy that may reduce sustainability rather than enhance it. By developing and implementing a suite of performance indicators, managers have the opportunity to manage toward a target level of a given indicator or predict the trend in the indicator over time. Developing, validating, and standardizing a set of sustainability indicators in animal agriculture has become a high research priority, and is vital, ironically, to the sustainability of the beef production chain in today's market environment.

DISCLOSURE

The author declares no external funding source and no conflicts of interest related to the preparation of this article.

REFERENCES

1. Goodland R, Daly H. Environmental sustainability: universal and non-negotiable. Ecol Appl 1996;6:1002–17.
2. World Commission on Environment and Development. Our common future. Oxford (UK): Oxford Univ. Press; 1987.
3. Meadows DH, Meadows DL, Randers J, et al. The limits to growth. New York: Universe Books; 1972.
4. Barbier EB. The concept of sustainable economic development. Environ Conserv 1987;14:101.
5. USDA, 2007. Sustainable agriculture: definitions and terms. Special Reference Brief no. SRB 99-02., Mary V. Gold, ed. Available at: http://www.nal.usda.gov/afsic/pubs/terms/srb9902.shtml.
6. Heitschmidt RK, Short RE, Grings EE. Ecosystems, sustainability, and animal agriculture. J Anim Sci 1996;74:1395–405.
7. Sterman J. Sustaining sustainability: creating a systems science in a fragmented academy and polarized world. In: Weinstein M, Turner RE, editors. Sustainability science: the emerging paradigm and the urban environment. Tokyo (Japan): Springer; 2012.
8. Costanza R, Patten BC. Defining and predicting sustainability. Ecol Econ 1995; 15:193–6.
9. Cabezas H, Pawlowski CW, Mayer AL, et al. Sustainable systems theory: ecological and other aspects. J Clean Prod 2005;5:455–67.
10. Purvis B, Mao Y, Robinson D. Sustainability Sci 2019;14:681–95.
11. Hirsch F. Social limits to growth. 2nd edition. London (United Kingdom): Routledge; 1995.
12. Searcy C. Corporate sustainability performance measurement systems: a review and research agenda. J Bus Ethics 2012;170:239–53.
13. Capper JL. The environmental impact of beef production in the United States: 1977 compared with 2007. J Anim Sci 2011;89:4249–61.
14. Rotz CA, Isenberg BJ, Stackhouse-Lawson KR, et al. A simulation-based approach for evaluating and comparing the environmental footprints of beef production systems. J Anim Sci 2013;91:5427–37.
15. Global Reporting Initiative. Sustainability reporting guidelines. Amsterdam (the Netherlands): Version 3.0. GRI; 2006.
16. Liverman DM, Hanson ME, Brown BJ, et al. Global sustainability: toward measurement. Environ Manag 1995;12:133–43.
17. Dale VH, Efroymson RA, Kline KL, et al. Indicators for assessing socioeconomic sustainability of bioenergy systems: A short list of practical measures. Ecol indicators 2013;26:87–102.
18. Baber JR, Sawyer JE, Wickersham TA. Estimation of human-edible protein conversion efficiency, net protein contribution, and enteric methane production from beef production in the United States. Translational Anim Sci 2018;2(4):439–50.
19. Davis K, Collins SR, Doty MM, Ho A, Holmgren A. 2005. Health and productivity among U.S. workers. Issue Brief (Commonw Fund) 2005 Aug;(856):1–10. PMID: 16138438.
20. Capper JL. Replacing rose-tinted spectacles with a high-powered microscope: the historical versus modern carbon footprint of animal agriculture. Anim Front 2011;1:26–32.

Using Mental Models to Improve Understanding of Cattle Diseases

Brian Vander Ley, DVM, PhD[a],*, John Dustin Loy, DVM, PhD[b],
Amelia R. Woolums, DVM, MVSc, PhD[c]

KEYWORDS

- Bovine disease • Systems thinking • Mental models

KEY POINTS

- Our understanding of how disease happens based on interpretation of observation and scientific discovery is a representation of reality, in other words, a mental model.
- All models, including mental models, are incomplete and require continuous adjustment and improvement to better represent reality.
- Inconsistencies between mental models of disease development and observations of disease discovery usually drive discoveries that improve our understanding of disease.

INTRODUCTION

Throughout history, the origins of disease have been studied to discover ways in which disease could be treated and prevented. For the discussion that follows, disease will be defined as the state in which one or more microbes create undesirable outcomes in a host (eg, pain, loss of function, loss of growth, death) as a result of an interaction with that host. This has been true for diseases of humans and animals. Understanding the origins of disease is closely tied to the cultural context and technological capabilities present at any particular point in time. Observation coupled with inductive reasoning led early physicians, scientists, and philosophers to formulate theories of disease based on associations. For example, Greek and Roman scholars linked diseases like malaria and fever with stagnant, swampy conditions.[1] Although one may be tempted to view such conclusions as archaic, these early observations demonstrate the

[a] University of Nebraska-Lincoln, School of Veterinary Medicine and Biomedical Sciences, Great Plains Veterinary Educational Center, PO Box 148, Clay Center, NE 68933, USA; [b] University of Nebraska-Lincoln, School of Veterinary Medicine and Biomedical Sciences, Nebraska Veterinary Diagnostic Center, 115Q NVDC, 4040 East Campus Loop N, Lincoln, NE 68583, USA; [c] Department of Pathobiology and Population Medicine, Mississippi State University, PO Box 6100, Starkville, MS 39762, USA
* Corresponding author.
E-mail address: bvanderley2@unl.edu

Vet Clin Food Anim 38 (2022) 219–227
https://doi.org/10.1016/j.cvfa.2022.02.004
0749-0720/22/© 2022 Elsevier Inc. All rights reserved.

power of developing accurate associations without uncovering true causation. Over time, these associative disease theories were refined and advanced through continued scholastic effort and technological advancements. Miasmas, contagion, and spontaneous generation all represent disease theories that evolved to account for inconsistencies with preceding theories. Equipped with the conception of germ theory put forth by Girolamo Fracastoro and the microscope invented by Anton von Leeuwenhoek, scientists like Francesco Redi and Louis Pasteur ushered in the golden age of microbiology.[1] With the contribution of his postulates, Robert Koch created a new framework to identify microbiological causes of disease.[2] Continuing advances in technology allowed scientists and medical practitioners to identify the causative agents in many disease processes. As advances were made in the understanding of how microbes caused disease and how the hosts responded to those microbes, new methods to control disease evolved. Veterinarians have participated in many of these efforts; for example, work by Daniel Salmon and the Bureau of Animal Industry that led to the eradication of contagious bovine pleuropneumonia in the United States in 1892.[3]

Microbes that fulfill Koch's postulates have been largely held in check by the development of antimicrobials, vaccines, and infection control. With the declining frequency and mitigated impacts of infectious diseases, other disease processes began to emerge that eluded fulfillment of Koch's postulates. In the 1980s, patients infected with the human immunodeficiency virus (HIV) suffered from life-threatening infections with microbes that had previously been considered innocuous to humans.[4] Because of the inconsistency of these types of infections with prevailing disease theory, Pirofski and Casadevall developed a new framework for understanding disease that would more fully account for clinical outcomes in their patients. This new framework is known as the damage–response framework (DRF).[5] The DRF provides a more complete explanation of the role of microbes and the host response in the production of disease.

A common theme running through history is the development of systems of thought designed to understand disease (ie, mental models). New observations, advancing technology, and developing thought adapt these mental models to resolve inconsistencies and improve the value of using the model. Observations by human and veterinary medical practitioners have played a central role in identifying inconsistencies in mental models of disease, without which technology and thought related to disease could not progress. The objectives of this article are to illustrate the progression of mental models relative to two common diseases of beef cattle and highlight important inconsistencies that are likely to be addressed in the next mental model of bovine disease.

BOVINE RESPIRATORY DISEASE

Bovine respiratory disease (BRD) of cattle is a prominent disease in cattle production systems in the United States and is the leading cause of illness and death in feedlot cattle.[6] BRD emerged as an economically relevant disease as US beef production began to rely more on transportation to capture regional advantages particular to the different production stages of cattle.[7] In fact, a common descriptive title for BRD is "shipping fever pneumonia." This designation appears frequently in the literature to describe respiratory disease occurring in calves following transport to feedlots. Over time, significant research efforts have been directed at understanding the etiology and pathogenesis of BRD. In the early to mid-twentieth century, veterinarians and scientists routinely published on the topic of BRD in journals like the *Journal of the American Veterinary Medical Association* and the *American Journal of Veterinary*

Research. In reviewing some of these publications, it is interesting to examine implicit and explicit assumptions about the disease being studied. Note that evaluating the assumptions of others is also based on the assumptions of the evaluator. As such, these evaluations are open to dialog and correction. In a report by Heath and Byrne, the authors conducted an experiment designed to determine whether "a virus or some other unrecognized agent" was associated with BRD in cattle by inoculating cattle, guinea pigs, and mice with cultures and tissue suspensions from diseased cattle.[8] The summary of their work states "Yearling cattle exposed by inhalation via the trachea, under the conditions described, were not visibly affected by the filtrate of infected lung tissue containing a few *Pasteurella*, by a pure culture of *Pasteurella*, or by a mixture of these inocula… The small infecting doses used might have had a bearing on the absence of visible symptoms." These authors are attempting to fulfill Koch's postulates for BRD but seem to believe they had failed in this case. Continued investigation into the etiology and pathogenesis of BRD in the 1970s and 1980s identified the pivotal role played by respiratory viruses in BRD development and attempted to control BRD through vaccination against these respiratory viruses.[9–11] Research in this arena led to the development of a "coinfection" mental model of disease where the development of bacterial bronchopneumonia was made possible by prior infection with a respiratory virus. Vaccination of calves at least once for respiratory viruses before leaving their birthplace has increased from 35.7% in 1997%–72.9% in 2017.[12,13] In the same approximate time frame, 14.4% of feedlot cattle were treated for BRD in 1999 compared with 16.2% in 2011.[14,15] These trends indicate that vaccination against respiratory viruses before sale is not directly causing a decrease in BRD occurrence in the feedlot. Although the coinfection model of disease certainly exists, manipulation of this model by vaccination against respiratory viruses has failed to produce the anticipated outcome of a reduction in BRD frequency. This unexpected outcome provides a strong indication that this model is inadequate to fully explain why BRD occurs.

A notable advancement in our model for BRD has arisen from the attention given to the host response. Research aimed at understanding immune function in cattle, including the impact of environment and management on immune function and the immune response to the microbes implicated in BRD, has provided proposed explanations for the inconsistencies of a model of disease based on coinfection with microbes alone. Several risk factors pertaining to management of cattle have been proposed and investigated. One commonly implicated risk factor was clearly delineated by the moniker "shipping fever." Livestock producers and veterinarians associated shipping events with the development of BRD in cattle. Transportation has been widely investigated as a risk factor for BRD with a range of outcomes. Taylor and colleagues reviewed proposed risk factors for BRD, including transport. In their review, the authors referred to reports that showed a mixture of effects associated with increasing transportation time or distance ranging from deleterious to insignificant.[16] After reviewing published evidence relating to many commonly held risk factors for BRD, Taylor and colleagues concluded that "A number of challenges exist that make effective field research of BRD difficult; nonetheless, existing knowledge does not provide sufficient support for many assertions that have become dogma in discussing BRD."[16]

Investigations of immune response to BRD have also been added to the model we use to understand BRD. A common understanding of increased risk for BRD was that susceptible calves had become immunocompromised by environmental and management factors. However, research evaluating the serum antibody responses of high-risk cattle vaccinated at feedlot arrival has demonstrated that these cattle can in fact be sufficiently immunocompetent to mount a humoral response to vaccination although vaccination at arrival has not been reliably related to decreased BRD morbidity in the weeks following vaccination.[17-19] The failure of vaccination to limit BRD in high-risk cattle that can mount an immune response to the vaccine could be the result of respiratory infection by agents not included in the vaccine. An alternative model that has been proposed is that BRD is the result of uncontrolled inflammation, and that cattle that resist BRD do so through successful modulation of inflammatory responses to bacteria that reach the lung.[20] This alternative model may mean that future efforts to limit BRD will be aimed less at killing bacteria and improving specific immunity to individual infectious agents classically associated with BRD and more at modulating inflammatory responses in cattle at risk for BRD.

The DRF mentioned in the introduction to this article may provide insight into ways that our mental model for BRD development might be enhanced. Like the physicians who conceptualized the DRF, veterinarians have been unable to effectively use a microbe-centric model of disease hinged on vaccination as the primary intervention to consistently modify BRD frequency in cattle. Similarly, consideration of the immune function of the calf without the context of a microbial infection fails to account for a necessary, but insufficient, cause of BRD in cattle. Perhaps an enhancement of our BRD mental model to include elements of the DRF may inspire a different view of BRD and how it could be controlled. Although not necessarily a new idea, an example of this change in view might be to consider the role of Mannheimia haemolytica or Histophilus somni given that both "pathogens" are routinely isolated from apparently healthy cattle and may even be useful in detecting pregnancy in cattle.[21]

INFECTIOUS BOVINE KERATOCONJUNCTIVITIS "BOVINE PINKEYE"

Similar to early work on BRD, infectious bovine keratoconjunctivitis (IBK) was a disease that had been described as "not a new disease by any means" by F.C. Billings in one of the first descriptions of IBK or "keratitis contagiosa" as it was described at the time.[22] Billings, a pathologist who had trained in the laboratories of Robert Koch and Rudolf Virchow, was the first University of Nebraska scientist devoted to full-time research, and through the Agricultural Experiment Station, was seeking to use Koch's framework to infectious diseases afflicting the livestock industries in the United States such as hog cholera and Texas Fever.[23] In his early description of IBK, he describes outbreaks of a disease, including illustrated figure panels, that most would immediately recognize as "pinkeye." Given his training in Koch's framework, Billings attempted to isolate and reproduce the disease and characterize the microorganisms responsible for the pathology. The microbes were observed in histologic sections and isolated and grown in pure culture from infected animals. Unsuccessful attempts were made to reproduce the disease in calves with scarified corneas. "No less remarkable has been the (in my experiments) absolute impossibility of intentional transmission of the disease from afflicted to healthy animals .... *the results were absolutely negative.*"[22]

This early work demonstrates in 1889 some of the challenges with direct application of Koch's framework in certain diseases. It is now better understood that Moraxella bovis (likely the same microorganisms observed by Dr Billings) can cause IBK, but it took another 70 years to convincingly reproduce the disease.[24] Other work has associated UV light, Mycoplasmas, and herpesviruses with outbreaks of this disease, sometimes in association with M bovis.[25-27] However, the ability to infect gnotobiotic calves with M bovis allowed full characterization of the pathology of the disease or at least a disease that clinically resembles descriptions of IBK.[28] Cell-free supernatants containing toxins produced by M bovis showed the ability to induce lesions consistent with IBK, demonstrating a specific toxin produced by M bovis may be causal.[29]

However, causality between Moraxella and IBK is not fully understood.[30] Other non-Moraxella agents have been implicated in the disease in some cases.[31] There is a great deal to be learned about environmental and other nonpathogen-associated risk factors that contribute to this disease, such as face flies, UV light, and dust that seem to have varying degrees of contribution to IBK.[32] Additionally, successful vaccination, a tactic that has been used broadly for numerous diseases since Koch, has been elusive for IBK. Maier and colleagues in a recent review state that "Despite 60 years of research into IBK vaccines, no effective vaccines appear to be widely available."[33] Given vaccines specifically target what is known about the pathogenesis of IBK, the multifactorial nature of the disease indicates that it would benefit from a re-examination of the model underlying it.

Another issue that complicates the study of IBK in a broader context or framework is the lack of a consistent case definition. This is a requirement for application to mental models and other understandings of diseases such as the DRF. Kneipp argues that IBK is used by veterinarians and producers as an "umbrella diagnosis" that lacks rigor and may hamper the ability to understand IBK more broadly.[34] Kneipp proposes a definition for IBK as "herd disease of cattle with high morbidity (mean proportion affected more than 2% in calves and 0.6% in cows) and rapid spread (mean time course within herd of 30 days) of clinical signs restricted to the eye, including conjunctivitis and/or keratitis with a significant number (10% or more) developing corneal ulceration."[34]

Implementation of an objective case definition combined with new mental models or disease frameworks may help to more fully realize the causality of IBK. DRF may be one conceptual model to consider (**Fig. 1**) where all environmental damage, host damage, and microbe/toxin damage contribute to elevating this damage to a level sufficient to cause disease. Depending on environmental and host factors, the risk for disease may be elevated under environmental or immunosuppressive conditions in addition to rapid circulation of toxin-secreting pathogens through vectors like face flies. When considering outbreaks at a population level, environmental factors such as dust and UV, fly vectors, and pathogen burden are herd-level factors rather than individual factors, thus promoting "outbreaks." The new case definition by Kneipp would account for measures of frequency (greater than 2%) and time (more than 30 days), in addition to a threshold level for clinical signs (10% or more with ulcers). This definition of disease reflects a significant change from thinking about disease as an individual condition to thinking about disease a condition of a population. Future investigation will certainly elucidate the value of this approach.

IMPLICATIONS FOR A SYSTEMS PRACTITIONER

Beef veterinarians face the task of applying the growing body of cattle disease knowledge to address the health challenges present in their clients' cattle. This task is particularly challenging when dissonance arises between scientific discoveries and observed outcomes. In this article, some of this information has been presented. For example, it may be surprising to some readers that despite an increase in vaccination of calves against the viruses associated with BRD before the movement of those calves into marketing channels, BRD incidence in feedlots has not been reduced.[12–15] This observation stands in contrast to a body of literature containing many well-designed experiments demonstrating the efficacy of BRD vaccines. A similar gap is also observed with IBK, where numerous experimental challenge studies demonstrate vaccine efficacy, but there is often a failure to observe this efficacy under field conditions.[33] For a veterinarian attempting to base

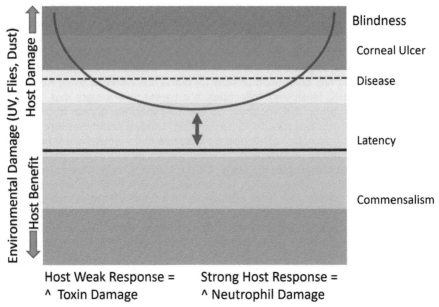

Fig. 1. Parabolic curve of the damage–response framework (Casadevall and Pirofski 2003) as applied to infectious bovine keratoconjunctivitis. The double-headed arrow indicates variation on the curve that is dependent on host–pathogen interaction. Host response is depicted on the *x*-axis and reflecting increased damage with either too weak of a response resulting in microbial toxin damage or too strong of a response resulting in neutrophil-related damage to ocular tissues. The *y*-axis (*left*) indicates contributions from the environment that alter host damage and benefit. The *y*-axis (*right*) indicates thresholds for disease to occur and the severity of disease outcomes.

recommendations on scientific evidence, this example creates dissonance that is difficult to resolve.

A basic tenet of systems thinking (ST) is that the structure of a system drives function that, in turn, produces outcomes. The developers of ST identified mental models as a foundation element in the structure of systems.[35] Although mental models are deeply personal and unique to individuals, groups of associated individuals often share many mental models. Models, including mental models, are useful representations of reality that serve as a basis for understanding. Conflict between existing mental models of disease and emerging scientific evidence usually indicates a flaw in the mental model, but that statement itself is a mental model.

Knowledge of beef cattle diseases is expanding as questions, new and old, are addressed from new vantage points with new technology. As each new discovery is revealed, it will be measured for fit in mental models of disease. There are at least two possible outcomes to this assessment of fit. First, the information may fit into an existing and well-accepted mental model that usually allows the information to be integrated easily. In other cases, the information may not fit the existing mental model leaving the evaluator with a choice of how best to integrate this information into existing paradigms. The information can be rejected outright to preserve the existing model or the model can be adapted to create an understanding that resolves, or lessens, the dissonance. In many cases, rejecting the information may be an appropriate response, as should be done if the information was invalid, lacked generalizability, or was confounded. The alternative is to accept the dissonant information and adapt the mental model to accommodate the new information in a best-fit approach.

Beef practitioners can provide critically important feedback in the process of improving mental models of disease in beef cattle. As strategies are developed to prevent or treat diseases in cattle, beef practitioners are often the first to view the results in the field and assess the outcomes. Perhaps an even more important role for beef practitioners is their long-term observations that highlight the discrepancy between the current understanding of disease and the outcomes in the field. These observations have been and will continue to be the impetus to refine the model with new questions and new approaches. Such new approaches will help to find new prevention solutions for diseases, especially complexes that likely have a complex causality. These models can be developed in an evidence-based manner to integrate new findings as they become available.

In the opinion of one of the authors (B.V.L.), increasing specialization has created fewer practitioners of medicine and research. Veterinarians caring for livestock have many demands on their time and resources that make participation in research challenges. Researchers face similar challenges that make clinical practice difficult to integrate with research activities. In each case, these conditions exist as a response to evolving circumstances. Examples presented in this article demonstrate the potential utility of the clinician and scientist being the same person as is the case with Drs Pirofski and Casadevall. Unfortunately, current indications point to increasing specialization. As a result, the need for communication between practitioners of medicine and practitioners of research will need to be robust. Communication of clinical impressions and objective measurements of disease from clinical practitioners to researchers will be vital in identifying inconsistencies in current models of disease. Similarly, communication from research practitioners to clinicians will be necessary to provide research results and the accompanying context of the mental models used to generate those results. Close collaboration will be necessary to allow all participants the opportunity to understand the structure of the systems in which they work more deeply.

CLINICS CARE POINTS

- Cattle veterinarians directly observe cattle diseases and are in a critical position to identify inconsistencies in mental models of disease.
- Cattle veterinarians can contribute to improved animal health by understanding existing models of disease, the assumptions included in those models, and communicating inconsistencies with the models.

DISCLOSURE

All authors have current or previous funding for bovine health research from public and private sources. One author (B.Vander Ley) has received honoraria to provide education on the topic of Systems Thinking to veterinarians.

REFERENCES

1. Karamanou M, Panayiotakopoulos G, Tsoucalas G, et al. From miasmas to germs: a historical approach to theories of infectious disease transmission. Le infezioni in medicina 2012;20(1):58–62.
2. Koch R. Über bakteriologische Forschung. Robert Koch-Institut; 2010.

3. Olmstead AL. The first line of defense: inventing the infrastructure to combat animal diseases. J Econ Hist 2009;69(2):327–57.

4. Pirofski L-a, Casadevall A. The damage–response framework as a tool for the physician-scientist to understand the pathogenesis of infectious diseases. J Infect Dis 2018;218(suppl_1):S7–11.

5. Casadevall A, Pirofski L-a. The damage-response framework of microbial pathogenesis. Nat Rev Microbiol 2003;1(1):17–24.

6. USDA. Feedlot 2011 "Part III: trends in health and management practices on U.S. Feedlots". Fort Collins (CO): USDA–APHIS–VS–CEAH, NAHMS; 2011.

7. Wilson LLM, K. G.; Mayo, H. H.; and Drewry, K. J., . "Development of the Beef Cattle Industry" Historical Documents of the Purdue Cooperative Extension Service. 1965;Paper 3.

8. Heath LM, Byrne JL. Shipping fever: i. search for a hypothetical agent associated with pasteurella. Can J Comp Med Vet Sci 1944;8(5):130–4.

9. Darcel CL, Jericho KW. Failure of a subunit bovine herpesvirus 1 vaccine to protect against experimental respiratory disease in calves. Can J Comp Med 1981; 45(1):87–91.

10. Jericho KW, Langford EV. Pneumonia in calves produced with aerosols of bovine herpesvirus 1 and Pasteurella haemolytica. Can J Comp Med 1978;42(3):269–77.

11. Jericho KW, Yates WD, Babiuk LA. Bovine herpesvirus-1 vaccination against experimental bovine herpesvirus-1 and Pasteurella haemolytica respiratory tract infection: onset of protection. Am J Vet Res 1982;43(10):1776–80.

12. USDA. NAHMS Beef 2017. 2017.

13. USDA. NAHMS Beef 2007. 2007.

14. USDA. NAHMS Feedlot 1999. 1999.

15. USDA. NAHMS Feedlot 2011. 2011.

16. Taylor JD, Fulton RW, Lehenbauer TW, et al. The epidemiology of bovine respiratory disease: what is the evidence for predisposing factors? Can Vet J 2010; 51(10):1095–102.

17. Griffin CM, Scott JA, Karisch BB, et al. A randomized controlled trial to test the effect of on-arrival vaccination and deworming on stocker cattle health and growth performance. Bovine Pract 2018;52(1):26–33.

18. Richeson JT, Beck PA, Gadberry MS, et al. Effects of on-arrival versus delayed modified live virus vaccination on health, performance, and serum infectious bovine rhinotracheitis titers of newly received beef calves. J Anim Sci 2008; 86(4):999–1005.

19. Richeson JT, Beck PA, Poe KD, et al. Effects of administration of a modified-live virus respiratory vaccine and timing of vaccination on health and performance of high-risk beef stocker calves. Bovine Pract 2015;49(1):37–42.

20. Bassel LL, Tabatabaei S, Caswell JL. Host tolerance to infection with the bacteria that cause bovine respiratory disease. Vet Clin North Am Food Anim Pract 2020; 36(2):349–59.

21. Deng F, McClure M, Rorie R, et al. The vaginal and fecal microbiomes are related to pregnancy status in beef heifers. J Anim Sci Biotechnol 2019;10(1):92.

22. Billings FS. Keratitis contagiosa in cattle. Nebr Agric Exp Station Bull 1889;10: 246–52.

23. Overfield RA. Hog Cholera, texas fever, and frank s billings: an episode in nebraska veterinary science. Nebr Hist 1976;57:29.

24. Henson JB, Grumbles LC. Infectious bovine keratoconjunctivitis. I. Etiology. Am J Vet Res 1960;21:761–6.

25. Hughes DE, Pugh GW Jr, McDonald TJ. Ultraviolet radiation and Moraxella bovis in the etiology of bovine infectious keratoconjunctivitis. Am J Vet Res 1965; 26(115):1331–8.
26. Rosenbusch RF. Influence of mycoplasma preinfection on the expression of Moraxella bovis pathogenicity. Am J Vet Res 1983;44(9):1621–4.
27. Pugh GW Jr, Hughes DE, Packer RA. Bovine infectious keratoconjunctivitis: interactions of Moraxella bovis and infectious bovine rhinotracheitis virus. Am J Vet Res 1970;31(4):653–62.
28. Rogers DG, Cheville NF, Pugh GW Jr. Pathogenesis of corneal lesions caused by Moraxella bovis in gnotobiotic calves. Vet Pathol 1987;24(4):287–95.
29. Beard MK, Moore LJ. Reproduction of bovine keratoconjunctivitis with a purified haemolytic and cytotoxic fraction of Moraxella bovis. Vet Microbiol 1994;42(1): 15–33.
30. Loy JD, Hille M, Maier G, et al. Component causes of infectious bovine keratoconjunctivitis - the role of moraxella species in the epidemiology of infectious bovine keratoconjunctivitis. Vet Clin North Am Food Anim Pract 2021;37(2):279–93.
31. Loy JD, Clothier KA, Maier G. Component causes of infectious bovine keratoconjunctivitis—non-moraxella organisms in the epidemiology of infectious bovine keratoconjunctivitis. Vet Clin North Am Food Anim Pract 2021;37(2):295–308.
32. Maier G, Doan B, O'Connor AM. The role of environmental factors in the epidemiology of infectious bovine keratoconjunctivitis. Vet Clin North Am Food Anim Pract 2021;37(2):309–20.
33. Maier G, O'Connor AM, Sheedy D. The evidence base for prevention of infectious bovine keratoconjunctivitis through vaccination. Vet Clin Food Anim Pract 2021; 37(2):341–53.
34. Kneipp M. Defining and diagnosing infectious bovine keratoconjunctivitis. Vet Clin North Am Food Anim Pract 2021;37(2):237–52.
35. Senge P. The Fifth Discipline: the art and practice of the learning organization. London (United Kingdom): Random House Books; 2006.

High-Risk Cattle Management and Stocker Calf Health

Modulation of the Bovine Respiratory Microbiome from a Systems Perspective

Brent Credille, DVM, PhD

KEYWORDS

- Bovine respiratory disease • Antimicrobial resistance • Microbiota
- *Mannheimia haemolytica* • *Pasteurella multocida*

KEY POINTS

- Bovine respiratory disease (BRD) is the most common cause of morbidity and mortality in North American beef cattle and affects animals across all industry segments.
- The US beef industry is diverse, broad, and segmented. The segmented nature of the beef industry results in the marketing of calves classified as high risk of developing BRD.
- The microbiota is the complex microbial ecosystem that exists in and on the body of all animals. The respiratory tract, like most other body systems, has its own unique microbiota that is shaped by many factors and evolves over the course of time. Importantly, the composition and diversity of the respiratory microbiota is believed to be associated with health and productivity and naturally begs the question, "How does manipulation of the microbiota influence respiratory tract health?"
- Modulation of the respiratory microbiota is an active area of investigation. Current modulation strategies rely on the use of antimicrobials. Unfortunately, antimicrobials disrupt beneficial bacterial community interactions and narrow the diversity of microorganisms in the respiratory tract. This potentially results in bacterial communities that are more permissive to colonization by opportunistic pathogens. Moreover, antimicrobial administration is associated with an increase in the abundance of antimicrobial resistance genes in respiratory tract samples.
- Health programs focused on the management of BRD in high-risk calves should be directed at the multiple components of the beef production system that disrupt the respiratory microbiota. Stress reduction, appropriate nutritional management, strategic use of vaccines, and antimicrobial administration targeted to the highest risk individuals all have the potential to stabilize an inherently unstable microbial population and enhance calf health.

Food Animal Health and Management Program, Department of Population Health, College of Veterinary Medicine, University of Georgia, Veterinary Medical Center, 2200 College Station Road, Athens, GA 30602, USA
E-mail address: Bc24@uga.edu

Vet Clin Food Anim 38 (2022) 229–243
https://doi.org/10.1016/j.cvfa.2022.03.001
0749-0720/22/© 2022 Elsevier Inc. All rights reserved.

INTRODUCTION

Bovine respiratory disease (BRD) is the most common and costly disease affecting beef cattle in North America. Within feedlots, BRD is responsible for approximately 75% of all morbidity and 50% of all mortality.[1] In stocker facilities, BRD occurs at a much greater frequency than what is commonly seen in feedlots and is estimated to be responsible for 90% of all morbidity and mortality in these operations.[2] Although multiple factors play a role in the development of BRD, bacterial pathogens are ultimately responsible for the clinical signs observed in affected cattle. The upper respiratory tract is likely the major reservoir of these opportunistic organisms, and, in the presence of stress or viral infections, they can proliferate, colonize the lower airway, and cause disease that results in significant economic losses and welfare compromise. There is an increasing amount of literature demonstrating the importance of a healthy microbiota to an animal's overall health and productivity.[3,4] Unfortunately, common practices associated with high-risk calf procurement and management have been shown to be disruptive to the establishment and maintenance of a healthy respiratory microbiota and predispose an animal to disease.[5] Extensive-drug antimicrobial resistance (XDR), or resistance to at least one antimicrobial agent in all but 1 or 2 classes, in clinically important BRD pathogens, as well as societal concerns regarding the use of medically important antimicrobials will, in the long term, serve to limit the availability and use of antimicrobials for treatment and control of BRD in high-risk cattle populations.[6–8] As a result, the development of nonantimicrobial methods of BRD control are desperately needed. Thus, the purpose of this article is to review the literature as it pertains to the respiratory microbiota, how factors inherent to high-risk calf production systems alter the respiratory microbiota and increase risk of BRD, as well as to provide an overview of how manipulation of the microbiota could improve cattle health and productivity.

STRUCTURE OF THE UNITED STATES BEEF INDUSTRY AND ROLE OF THE STOCKER SEGMENT

The beef cattle industry is a diverse and important contributor to the US economy. Today, approximately 619,000 beef cattle operations and 30 million beef cows are currently in the United States. Interestingly, it is estimated that 90% of cow-calf operations have less than 100 head of cattle with these operations representing nearly 50% of the total US cattle population. Moreover, the average cattle producer in the United States has a herd that is made up of 40 or fewer head of cattle and current estimates indicate the economic impact of these operations and the cattle on them exceeds $88 billion yearly.[9]

Although often seen as a single entity, the North American beef industry is divided into multiple distinct segments and each segment operates with different management focuses and different end goals in mind (**Fig. 1**). One critically important segment of the beef industry is the stocker segment, as stockers represent a link between cow-calf producers and cattle feeders and approximately 74% of calves will end up spending some amount of time in a stocker facility before entering a feedlot. Cow-calf operations market calves on a semiseasonal schedule with most calves being marketed in the early to late fall.[10] Cattle feeding, however, is constant throughout the course of the year so that the needs of the industry and consumer can effectively be met. Stocker operations play a critical role in managing this seasonal and irregular supply of feeder cattle and can buffer both excess and inadequate animal availability.[11,12] Unfortunately, many feeder calves born to cow-calf producers in the United States are not suitable for movement directly to feed yards at the time of marketing. Cultural and economic factors often result in

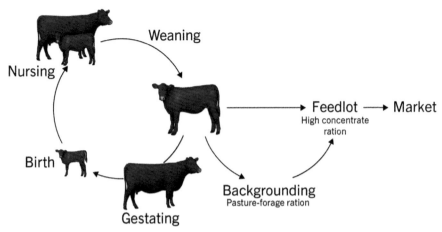

Fig. 1. Structure of the North American beef cattle production system and flow of cattle from segment to segment.

cow-calf producers marketing calves before they are adequately prepared for finishing.[10] As a result, cattle arriving at stocker facilities are purchased in small lots, lightweight and in poor nutritional status, unweaned, and of unknown health status (ie, unvaccinated, not dewormed). In addition, these cattle are often commingled with cattle from multiple other sources, and males are left intact. Sometimes, cattle are transported long distances without regular access to feed and water, suffer from dehydration and enter into a negative energy balance.[13] Stocker enterprises manage these high-risk calves to improve their health and add weight, sort them into groups of uniform size, weight, and color, and market them to feedlots as a value-added product.[11] These types of operations ensure a constant supply of feeder cattle to enter feedlots. Thus, without stocker facilities, many US cattle producers would have little to no potential to market their cattle in a cost-effective manner and many cow-calf operations would struggle to make ends meet. As a result, stockers are a significant contributor to the US economy and the sustainability of the US beef industry.[14] Thus, the stocker/backgrounder segment provides a way for cow-calf producers to remain viable, and competitive, in the modern beef industry.[14]

Unfortunately, the very factors that make stocker operations an integral component of the beef industry also dramatically increase the risk that a high proportion of calves will develop BRD. For example, commingling and lack of weaning have been shown to increase the risk of BRD relative to single-source and preconditioned calves significantly.[15,16] In addition, bulls, because they are likely to be castrated during or immediately after arrival, are significantly more likely to develop and succumb to the effects of BRD.[17] Currently, the only consistently effective tool for managing high-risk calf health is metaphylaxis, and the long-term sustainability of this technology is in question because of public perception of antimicrobial use in animal agriculture and the increased prevalence of XDR bacterial isolates in relevant cattle populations.[18,19]

THE MICROBIOME AND THE RESPIRATORY TRACT: FROM DEVELOPMENT TO DISEASE
A Historical Perspective and Overview of Factors Affecting the Development of the Respiratory Microbiota in Healthy Cattle

The use of the term microbiome was standardized in the early 21st century and defined as the community of all microorganisms (bacteria, fungi, viruses, etc) living within a specific environmental niche.[20] In the case of mammals, this term is used to describe all members of the microbiota, as well as their genomic material and the surrounding environment. The normal structure of the microbiota is organ specific, with each body site and organ system having its own specific microbiota.[20] To date, much of the work describing the microbiota of the healthy and diseased bovine respiratory tract has been focused on bacterial agents and comparatively little is known about the contribution of viruses, fungi, and phages.[4,21,22] As a result, much of the following discussion is largely limited to bacteria.

Historically, the lungs were thought to be sterile and free from any and all bacterial colonization.[20] This misconception was based on limitations of available laboratory techniques. Advances in next-generation sequencing technologies have provided a window into the composition and function of the resident microbiota of the mammalian body.[23] Today, it is known that even the lungs of healthy people and animals harbor bacteria. In people, for example, the lungs of clinically healthy adults contain between 10^3 to 10^5 bacteria per gram of tissue. Moreover, these microbial communities have coevolved with their host to occupy a particular niche and play a significant role in the promotion and maintenance of health.[23]

The development of the respiratory microbiota begins early in life. In cattle, colonization of the respiratory tract starts at parturition and is heavily influenced by maternal vaginal microbiota, ingestion of colostrum, antimicrobial administration, and housing/environmental conditions present at the time of birth.[24] It is likely that early microbial composition of the respiratory tract influences both the structure of the microbiota and respiratory health later in life. Indeed, work in people has shown that ingestion of high-quality colostrum promotes the development of a microbiota that is associated with a reduction in the risk of respiratory infections later in childhood. Moreover, factors such as method of delivery, feeding routines (formula vs nursing), crowding, and antimicrobial administration have all been shown to be associated with alterations in the respiratory microbiota and an increased risk of respiratory tract infections later in life. In newborn calves, heat treatment of colostrum collected from dairy cattle and fed to newborn calves is associated with a reduction in the early colonization of the gut with Escherichia coli, increased levels of Bifidobacterium spp, and a reduced likelihood for treatment of both diarrhea and respiratory disease in the preweaning phase of growth. Work in dairy calves has shown that the total bacterial load in the upper respiratory tract at day 3 of life was higher in calves that developed pneumonia than those that remained healthy.[24,25] In addition, this same study showed that calves born to dams that harbored Mannheimia in their vagina were significantly less likely to get sick than calves born to dams that did not harbor Mannheimia.[24] It is likely that these early colonizers stimulate immune responses that carry through early life and reflect the induction of antigen-specific immune responses at mucosal surfaces. Finally, as an example of how potentially negative influences on the microbiota can shape calf health, a study found that administration of tulathromycin to Holstein calves within the first 12 hours of life was associated with greater numbers of E coli in the feces on days 20 to 23 after birth, a higher incidence of diarrhea in the first 2 weeks of life, and suppression in neutrophil function relative to untreated animals.[26]

Structure and Composition of the Respiratory Microbiota in Healthy Cattle

The mucosal surfaces of the upper and lower airways harbor diverse and distinct microbial communities. Differences in environmental exposures, pH, P_{CO_2}, temperature, epithelial cell type, and immune status all interact to select for a specific pattern of microbial growth. The microbiota of the upper respiratory tract has, to date, been the best characterized and it has been shown that the nasopharyngeal (NP) microbiota is composed of bacteria from more than 29 different phyla and 300 different genera.[3] Despite this wealth of diversity, 5 bacterial phyla, namely the Proteobacteria, Firmicutes, Tenericutes, Actinobacteria, and Bacteroidetes, are known to make up much of the NP respiratory microbiota in the healthy animal, with organisms within the phyla Actinobacteria and Proteobacteria being most abundant and least abundant, respectively (**Table 1**).[3] Within these phyla, bacteria from the genera *Corynebacterium, Moraxella, Mycoplasma, Pasteurella, Mannheimia, Psychrobacter,* and *Staphylococcus* are the most common and abundant. In the lower respiratory tract (ie, trachea and lung) of healthy cattle, organisms in the phyla Tenericutes, Firmicutes, Proteobacteria, and Bacteriodetes are enriched relative to others. Within these 4 phyla, bacteria from the genera *Mycoplasma, Streptomyces, Streptococcus, Mannheimia,* and *Moraxella* are most abundant.[3] Although it is generally accepted that the NP is the source of bacteria for the lower airway, this has never been definitively proven and remains somewhat controversial. In people, for example, bacteria reaching the lower airway originate from the mouth and oropharynx.[20] However, more recent work evaluating the topography of the respiratory microbiota in healthy feedlot cattle found that the microbiota of the lung is most like the microbiota of the NP and confirmed that the NP is, indeed, the likely source for bacteria found in the lung of both healthy and diseased cattle and studies characterizing the NP microbiota also do an adequate job of characterizing the microbiota of the lower airway.[21] It is important to note that, despite attempts to characterize a normal microbiota, there is much variability in NP microbiota composition between groups and within individual cattle in a group.[3]

The respiratory microbiome and lung homeostasis

Although most studies on the respiratory microbiota in healthy cattle have focused on community structure, it is clear from other species that specific microbial populations are important to maintaining respiratory homeostasis. More specifically, the normal microbial population of the respiratory tract is important in modulating host immune defenses. In addition, microbiota/immune crosstalk, the phenomenon by which alterations in bacterial populations impact local and systemic immunity, is essential for regulating mucosal immune responses.[27] This modulation can be done in multiple different ways. First, members of the normal respiratory microbiota can compete with pathogenic organisms for nutrients, adhesion sites, and receptors within a specific niche.[27] Second, respiratory commensals produce inhibitory compounds such

Table 1 Specific bacterial phyla and genera associated with the nasopharyngeal microbiota in healthy cattle	
Phyla	**Characteristics and Examples of Organisms within Phyla**
Proteobacteria	Largest phylum within bacterial domain; Gram (−) staining and lipopolysaccharide in outer cell wall (*Mannheimia, Pasteurella, Histophilus*)
Firmicutes	Gram (+) cell wall structure with low guanine-cytosine content in genome (*Lactobacilli* and *Clostridiales*)
Tenericutes	Small prokaryotic organisms that lack a cell wall (*Mycoplasma* and *Ureaplasma*)
Actinobacteria	Gram (+) cell wall structure with high guanine-cytosine content in genome (*Bifidobacterium* and *Actinomyces*)
Bacteroidetes	Gram (−) cell wall structure and non–spore-forming (*Bacteroides* and *Prevotella*)

as hydrogen peroxide and lactic acid that are toxic to pathogenic microbes.[27] Lastly, normal bacteria have a potent immunomodulatory role.[27] In mouse models, for example, colonization of the lung with Bacteroidetes has been shown to decrease lung inflammation relative to colonization with other organisms.[28] In addition, bacteria known to be part of the normal microbiota have been shown to recruit monocytes to the lungs and stimulate their differentiation into immunosuppressive macrophages.[29] These macrophages dampen inflammatory responses to infection with pathogenic viruses and bacteria.[29] Also, the normal microbiota is essential for the recruitment of dendritic cells to the lungs.[30] These dendritic cells crosstalk with T cells and stimulate the release of IgA at the respiratory mucosal surface.[23,30] The secreted IgA prevents pathogenic organisms from interacting with the respiratory epithelium and selects for expansion of a healthy and more heterogeneous microbiota (**Fig. 2**).[23]

Factors Affecting the Respiratory Microbiome in High-Risk Calves

Typically, the clinical signs of BRD are associated with colonization of the lower airway by limited numbers of virulent bacterial pathogens, namely Mannheimia *haemolytica*, Pasteurella *multocida*, *Histophilus somni*, and *Mycoplasma bovis*.[31] As a result of this

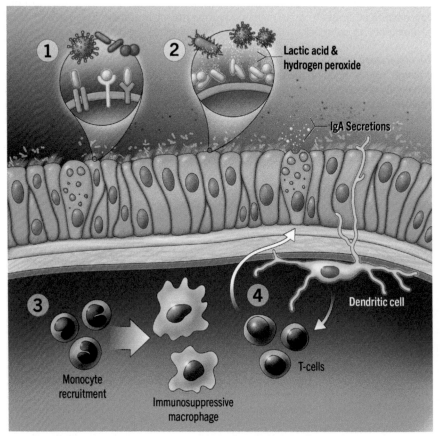

Fig. 2. Mechanisms by which the microbiota control colonization of the airway with pathogenic microorganisms.

limited focus, our therapeutic efforts have been aimed at controlling the overgrowth of these pathogens in the lower airway with antimicrobials. These common pathogens, however, are often commensal residents of the NP and, in conjunction with other bacteria, fungi, and viruses, form elaborate ecological networks.[32] At equilibrium, these networks prime the host immune system and prevent colonization with virulent microbes.[3] When these networks are disturbed, bacterial overgrowth develops and disease results. The very nature of stocker production systems predisposes to ecological perturbations in the NP microbiota and these perturbations impair immune function, negatively affect colonization resistance, and predispose to bacterial overgrowth and clinical BRD.[5] Thus, the focus of our preventive efforts, at least in the context of the microbiota, should be to minimize the impact of the various stressful events a calf experiences so that the structure of the "healthy" microbiota is maintained.

It is important to understand that the composition of the respiratory microbiota evolves over time and is influenced by multiple factors. For example, the temperature, moisture, and pH of the respiratory mucosa promote the growth of some and limit the growth of other organisms.[3] In addition, exogenous forces such as diet, health status, stress (ie, weaning, transport, commingling), and antimicrobial administration have a profound influence on the structure and composition of the respiratory microbiota (**Fig. 3**).[4,33] In high-risk populations of beef cattle, the normal processes associated with procurement and processing these animals serve as a major deterrent to the maintenance of a healthy microbiota and predispose these animals to the development of BRD.

Weaning, commingling, and dietary influences
Between leaving the farm of origin and the first week in a feedlot, the diversity of the NP microbiota increases dramatically, with approximate doubling in the number of bacterial taxons identified in that time frame.[5,34] Within approximately 45 to 60 days, however, the shifts in NP microbiota stabilize and the bacterial populations

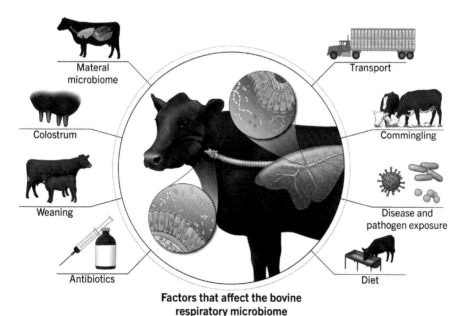

Material microbiome

Colostrum

Weaning

Antibiotics

Transport

Commingling

Disease and pathogen exposure

Diet

Factors that affect the bovine respiratory microbiome

Fig. 3. Factors affecting the structure of the respiratory microbiota in cattle.

of the NP become more homogenous.[34] Indeed, at the time of arrival, organisms within the phyla Proteobacteria and Firmicutes dominate with bacteria in the genera *Pseudomonas, Shewanella,* and *Acinetobacter* being most prevalent. By day 60, however, organisms within the phyla Tenericutes increase in prevalence with bacteria in the genera *Staphylococcus, Mannheimia, Moraxella,* and *Mycoplasma* being most common (**Fig. 4**).[34] These shifts can be explained by transportation and exposure to a new environment with a preponderance of animals from different cattle operations. Moreover, changes in diet, environment, geographic location, and conspecific exposure also likely contribute to alterations in the respiratory microbiota.[3] In the context of commingling, however, a minimum duration and frequency of contact is needed before changes in the NP microbiota occur.[5] Work has shown that 24 hours of exposure at an auction market was not sufficient to affect the diversity of the NP microbiota in 2 groups of weaned beef calves.[5] More recent work performed in 6-month-old beef calves subjected to an experimental model of weaning and transport stress found that stressed calves had an increase in the abundance of Tenericutes and Bacteroidetes and a decrease in the abundance of Proteobacteria in the NP relative to unstressed, nursing calves.[35] Moreover, these changes in the NP microbiota began to occur within 2 days of the stressful event and continued to evolve over the course of the 28-day sampling period.[35] Additional work in cattle raised without antimicrobials has shown that, as the number of days on feed (DOF) progresses, the variation in NP microbiota changes.[22] Most notable is the finding that *M bovis* increases in abundance as the number of DOF increases. This suggests stocker and feedlot operations may serve as a reservoir of this organism and contagious spread of this organism occurs between animals in a specific environment.[22] Similarly, work evaluating the gastrointestinal microbiome in feedlot cattle found that number of DOF better explained the variation seen in the fecal microbiota than did other factors analyzed.[36]

Vaccination
Relatively little is known about the impact of vaccination on the NP microbiota. Nevertheless, recent work has shown that the administration of an intranasal modified live

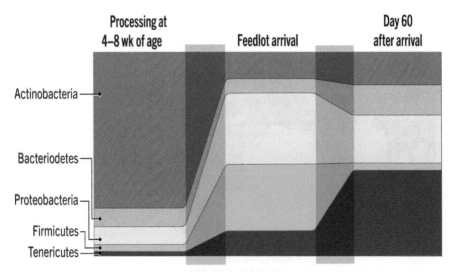

Fig. 4. Changes in the structure of the respiratory microbiota from nursing through 60 days after feedlot arrival.

viral vaccine to nursing Holstein calves increased the mucosal IgA response to both *M haemolytica* and *P multocida.*[37] Although the reasons for the increase in titer and the significance of this finding to respiratory health are not clear, it is possible that this response might be more harmful than beneficial, as administration of vaccine to these calves could be associated with rapid proliferation of these organisms in the upper airway. In the right animal, this overgrowth of bacteria could increase, rather than decrease, the risk of disease occurring. Similarly, work in human models has found that the type I interferon response induced by the administration of attenuated live intranasal influenza vaccines (LAIV) permitted greater persistence of potentially pathogenic strains of *Staphylococcus aureus.*[38] In addition, LAIV have been shown to increase pneumococcal density in the upper airway of vaccine recipients.[39] Although not considered an issue for healthy recipients within a population, this increased pathogen density has been shown to increase pneumococcal transmission and prevalence and increase disease risk in the most susceptible within a group.[39,40] In cattle, recent work has shown that vaccine administration to high-risk calves has, at best, little impact on risk of BRD and, at worst, a negative effect on animal health and welfare.[41–44] As a result, studies evaluating the impact of vaccine administration on the respiratory microbiota and the role of any perturbations in the respiratory microbiota on calf health are needed.

Health status

BRD is a multifactorial disease syndrome associated with colonization of the upper and lower airways with viral and bacterial pathogens.[2] It is generally accepted that viral damage to the respiratory tract precedes colonization with virulent bacteria.[45] In chinchillas, experimental infection with respiratory syncytial virus (RSV) has been shown to alter the expression of acute-phase proteins in the NP and promote overgrowth of *Haemophilus influenzae.*[46] In addition, work in human infants has shown that RSV infection increases the relative amounts of cytokines associated with antiviral and proinflammatory activities and that these cytokines promote an environment permissive to overgrowth of common respiratory pathogens.[47,48] BRD has a significant impact on the makeup of the upper and lower respiratory tract microbiota.[22] More specifically, most studies have found that cattle diagnosed with BRD have a significant decrease in richness and abundance in the NP microbiota when compared with healthy cattle.[22] Cattle diagnosed with BRD have greater abundances of Tenericutes and Proteobacteria and a decreased abundance of Firmicutes when compared with healthy cattle. At the level of specific genera, cattle with BRD have greater abundances of *M bovis, Bacteroides, Histophilus, Mannheimia, Moraxella,* and *Fusobacterium* and decreased abundances of *Mycoplasma dispar, Lactococcus, Corynebacterium,* and *Akkermansia.* In a study that evaluated changes in the NP microbiota in 135 single source Charolais calves, a diagnosis of BRD was found to be associated with an increase in the proportion of *Acinetobacter* spp, *Solibacillus* spp, and *Pasteurella* spp.[49] A Canadian study found that organisms such as *M bovis, P multocida,* and *M haemolytica* are found more often in the NP and trachea of feedlot cattle with BRD when compared with healthy cattle.[50] Work in cattle raised without antimicrobials found cattle diagnosed with BRD had a significant increase in the proportion of samples with *Mycoplasma bovis/agalactiae* and *Mycoplasma bovirhinis,* as well as a tendency toward increased numbers of *H somni* and *Mannheimia* spp.[22] In contrast, the lungs of feedlot cattle that remain healthy have a greater abundance of *Micrococcaceae* and *Lachnospiraceae* at arrival and 60 days later, respectively, when compared with cattle that develop BRD.[22] Moreover, the relative abundance of both *Lactobacillaceae* and *Bacillaceae* is greater in the NP of cattle that remain healthy when compared with animals subsequently diagnosed with BRD. Interestingly, the *Lactobacillaceae* family includes bacteria in the genera *Lactobacillus* and *Pediococcus* and specific species within these genera have been associated with a decrease in the shedding of *E coli 0157:H7* in feedlot cattle.[51] In addition, studies have shown that the *Lactobacilli* inhibit in vitro growth and reduce nasal colonization with *M haemolytica* through a combination of displacement, competition, and immunomodulation.[51,52]

Antimicrobial administration

The use of antimicrobials has revolutionized our ability to manage BRD in high-risk populations of cattle.[18] Unfortunately, concerns over the increasing prevalence of resistance in common BRD pathogens and our improved understanding of the role of a healthy microbiota on respiratory health are forcing a closer look at accepted antimicrobial use strategies and how they impact the microbiota and subsequent disease risk.[2,3,19] For example, parenteral administration of antimicrobials for the treatment or control of BRD in high-risk populations of cattle disrupt microbial community interactions and this makes these communities more permissive to colonization by pathogenic microbes.[53] Experimental models have shown that exposure of *Vibrio cholerae* to tetracycline alters the structure of bacterial biofilms, making them more permissive to invasion by phages and bacterial cells of different species that would usually be unable to do so.[54] Mass medication of high-risk cattle with tulathromycin, enrofloxacin, and tildipirosin has been associated with the contagious spread of *M haemolytica* strains that harbor an integrative conjugative element harboring genes that confer resistance to multiple different antimicrobials.[6,8,55,56] In a study evaluating the impact of either oxytetracycline or tulathromycin administration on the microbiota of feedlot considered to be at high risk of developing BRD, antimicrobial administration was found to have long-lasting (>60 days) impacts on the NP microbiota.[53] More specifically, cattle given either antimicrobial had significant greater abundances of *Pseudomonas*, *Paeniglutamicibacter*, and *Camobacterium* than cattle that received only chlortetracycline in feed.[53] Moreover, when compared with entry samples, cattle that received either oxytetracycline or tulathromycin had reduced abundances of *Mannheimia*, *Mycoplasma,* and *Pasteurella* at feedlot exit when compared with cattle receiving only in-feed chlortetracycline. In another study evaluating the longitudinal effects of either oxytetracycline or tulathromycin on the fecal and respiratory microbiota of single-source feedlot cattle, the administration of oxytetracycline resulted in disturbances to the microbiota that lasted for a longer period (>35 days) when compared with cattle given tulathromycin.[57] In cattle that received tulathromycin, the NP microbiota returned to baseline by day 12 postantimicrobial administration.[57] In addition, even though oxytetracycline administration was associated with an initial decrease in the abundance of *Mycoplasma* spp in the NP, this quickly shifted and oxytetracycline administration was associated with an increase in *Mycoplasma* spp later in the feeding period. In addition, the administration of both oxytetracycline and tulathromycin was associated with an increase in the abundance of multiple different antimicrobial resistance genes.[57] More recently, work evaluating the impact of a single dose of tilmicosin at the time of BRD diagnosis found that tilmicosin had little impact on the NP microbiota and treated animals had an NP microbiota that more closely resembled that of animals with BRD when compared with healthy controls.[58] Indeed, cattle treated with tilmicosin had an increased abundance of Firmicutes and a decreased abundance of Proteobacteria when compared with pretreatment samples.[58] At the genus level, tilmicosin-treated cattle had an increase in the abundance of *Acinetobacter*, *Lachnospiraceae,* and *Clostridium* and a decrease in the abundance of

Turicibacter and *Microbacteriacease* compared with healthy controls.[58] Overall, the administration of tilmicosin to cattle with BRD was associated with minor changes in the NP microbiota when compared with healthy control cattle and the NP microbiota of treated calves more closely resembled that of BRD-affected animals.[58] It is important to note, however, that this work had no untreated controls and involved relatively small numbers of animals. As a result, it may have the potential to be overinterpreted and more data are needed before more definitive conclusions can be drawn.

SUMMARY

The structure of the North American beef cattle production system is conducive to the marketing of cattle that are considered to be at high risk for the development of BRD. The microbiota is the population of microorganisms that live within and on the various body systems of mammals and the composition of the microbiota is associated with health and productivity. The development of a "healthy" respiratory microbiota begins as early as the first day of life and factors inherent to high-risk cattle production systems (commingling, transport, lack of weaning, and health history) result in further disruption to the microbiota of the upper and lower respiratory tract. In addition, common stocker management practices (vaccination and metaphylaxis) likely worsen the perturbations occurring within an already unstable microbiota and further increase disease susceptibility or predispose to the selection of antimicrobial-resistant strains of bacteria. Optimization of respiratory tract health and maintenance of a normal microbiota is dependent on multiple factors that begin on the cow-calf operation and continue to be susceptible to alteration through the first 60 days after arrival to a feedlot or stocker facility. Modulation of the microbiota through administration of probiotics or improved calf management practices has the potential to enhance calf health and improve the overall sustainability of the entire beef production system.

CLINICS CARE POINTS

- Although often associated with a limited number of virulent viral and bacterial pathogens, bovine respiratory disease (BRD) actually reflects a disturbance in the respiratory microbiota.

- Prevention of BRD should be focused on limiting management procedures and therapeutic interventions that disrupt a "healthy" respiratory microbiota.

- Maintenance of a healthy microbiota through a rethinking of how beef cattle are managed can improve calf health and the overall sustainability of the modern beef production system.

DISCLOSURE

The author has nothing to disclose.

REFERENCES

1. Aphis U. Feedlot 2011 Part IV: health and health management on U.S. Feedlots with a capacity of 1,000 or more head 2013. 27-45.
2. Snyder E, Credille B. *Mannheimia haemolytica* and *Pasteurella multocida* in bovine respiratory disease: how are they changing in response to efforts to control them? Vet Clin North Am Food Anim Pract 2020;36:253–68.

3. Timsit E, McMullen C, Amat S, et al. Respiratory bacterial microbiota in cattle: from development to modulation to enhance respiratory health. Vet Clin North Am Food Anim Pract 2020;36:297–320.

4. Alexander TW, Timsit E, Amat S. The role of the bovine respiratory bacterial microbiota in health and disease. Anim Health Res Rev 2020;21:168–71.

5. Stroebel C, Alexander T, Workentine ML, et al. Effects of transportation to and comingling at an auction market on nasopharyngeal and tracheal bacterial communities of recently weaned beef cattle. Vet Microbiol 2018;223:126–33.

6. Woolums AR, Karisch BB, Frye JG, et al. Multidrug resistant *Mannheimia haemolytica* isolated from high-risk beef stocker cattle after antimicrobial metaphylaxis and treatment for bovine respiratory disease. Vet Microbiol 2018;221:143–52.

7. Lubbers BV, Hanzlicek GA. Antimicrobial multidrug resistance and coresistance patterns of *Mannheimia haemolytica* isolated from bovine respiratory disease cases–a three-year (2009-2011) retrospective analysis. J Vet Diagn Invest 2013;25:413–7.

8. Snyder E, Credille B, Berghaus R, et al. Prevalence of multi drug antimicrobial resistance in *Mannheimia haemolytica* isolated from high-risk stocker cattle at arrival and two weeks after processing. J Anim Sci 2017;95:1124–31.

9. Drouillard JS. Current situation and future trends for beef production in the United States of America - A review. Asian-Australas J Anim Sci 2018;31:1007–16.

10. Groves JT. Details to attend to when managing high-risk cattle. Vet Clin North Am Food Anim Pract 2020;36:445–60.

11. Peel DS. Economics of stocker production. Vet Clin North Am Food Anim Pract 2006;22:271–96.

12. Peel DS. Beef cattle growing and backgrounding programs. Vet Clin North Am Food Anim Pract 2003;19:365–85, vi.

13. Adkins ML, Rollin E, Heins BD, et al. Evaluation of serum metabolic parameters as predictors of bovine respiratory disease events in high-risk beef stocker calves. Bovine Pract 2020;54:9–16.

14. Peel DS. Economic considerations of enhanced BRD control. Anim Health Res Rev 2020;21:139–42.

15. Step DL, Krehbiel CR, DePra HA, et al. Effects of commingling beef calves from different sources and weaning protocols during a forty-two-day receiving period on performance and bovine respiratory disease. J Anim Sci 2008;86:3146–58.

16. Wilson BK, Richards CJ, Step DL, et al. Best management practices for newly weaned calves for improved health and well-being. J Anim Sci 2017;95:2170–82.

17. Richeson JT, Pinedo PJ, Kegley EB, et al. Association of hematologic variables and castration status at the time of arrival at a research facility with the risk of bovine respiratory disease in beef calves. J Am Vet Med Assoc 2013;243: 1035–41.

18. Nickell JS, White BJ. Metaphylactic antimicrobial therapy for bovine respiratory disease in stocker and feedlot cattle. Vet Clin North Am Food Anim Pract 2010; 26:285–301.

19. Credille B. Antimicrobial resistance in *Mannheimia haemolytica*: prevalence and impact. Anim Health Res Rev 2020;21:196–9.

20. Wypych TP, Wickramasinghe LC, Marsland BJ. The influence of the microbiome on respiratory health. Nat Immunol 2019;20:1279–90.

21. McMullen C, Alexander TW, Léguillette R, et al. Topography of the respiratory tract bacterial microbiota in cattle. Microbiome 2020;8:91.

22. McMullen C, Orsel K, Alexander TW, et al. Comparison of the nasopharyngeal bacterial microbiota of beef calves raised without the use of antimicrobials

between healthy calves and those diagnosed with bovine respiratory disease. Vet Microbiol 2019;231:56–62.

23. Man WH, de Steenhuijsen Piters WA, Bogaert D. The microbiota of the respiratory tract: gatekeeper to respiratory health. Nat Rev Microbiol 2017;15:259–70.

24. Lima SF, Bicalho MLS, Bicalho RC. The *Bos taurus* maternal microbiome: role in determining the progeny early-life upper respiratory tract microbiome and health. PLoS One 2019;14:e0208014.

25. Lima SF, Teixeira AG, Higgins CH, et al. The upper respiratory tract microbiome and its potential role in bovine respiratory disease and otitis media. Sci Rep 2016; 6:29050.

26. Martin CC, Baccili CC, Avila-Campos MJ, et al. Effect of prophylactic use of tula-thromycin on gut bacterial populations, inflammatory profile and diarrhea in newborn Holstein calves. Res Vet Sci 2021;136:268–76.

27. van den Broek MFL, De Boeck I, Kiekens F, et al. Translating recent microbiome insights in otitis media into probiotic strategies. Clin Microbiol Rev 2019;32.

28. Donaldson GP, Ladinsky MS, Yu KB, et al. Gut microbiota utilize immunoglobulin A for mucosal colonization. Science 2018;360:795–800.

29. Wang J, Li F, Sun R, et al. Bacterial colonization dampens influenza-mediated acute lung injury via induction of M2 alveolar macrophages. Nat Commun 2013;4:2106.

30. Herbst T, Sichelstiel A, Schär C, et al. Dysregulation of allergic airway inflamma-tion in the absence of microbial colonization. Am J Respir Crit Care Med 2011; 184:198–205.

31. Timsit E, Hallewell J, Booker C, et al. Prevalence and antimicrobial susceptibility of *Mannheimia haemolytica, Pasteurella multocida, and Histophilus somni* iso-lated from the lower respiratory tract of healthy feedlot cattle and those diag-nosed with bovine respiratory disease. Vet Microbiol 2017;208:118–25.

32. Timsit E, Workentine M, van der Meer F, et al. Distinct bacterial metacommunities inhabit the upper and lower respiratory tracts of healthy feedlot cattle and those diagnosed with bronchopneumonia. Vet Microbiol 2018;221:105–13.

33. Hall JA, Isaiah A, Bobe G, et al. Feeding selenium-biofortified alfalfa hay during the preconditioning period improves growth, carcass weight, and nasal microbial diversity of beef calves. PLoS One 2020;15:e0242771.

34. McMullen C, Orsel K, Alexander TW, et al. Evolution of the nasopharyngeal bac-terial microbiota of beef calves from spring processing to 40 days after feedlot arrival. Vet Microbiol 2018;225:139–48.

35. Malmuthuge N, Howell A, Arsic N, et al. Effect of maternal separation and trans-portation stress on the bovine upper respiratory tract microbiome and the im-mune response to resident opportunistic pathogens. Anim Microbiome 2021; 3:62.

36. Doster E, Rovira P, Noyes NR, et al. Investigating effects of tulathromycin meta-phylaxis on the fecal resistome and microbiome of commercial feedlot cattle early in the feeding period. Front Microbiol 2018;9:1715.

37. Midla LT, Hill KL, Van Engen NK, et al. Innate and acquired immune responses of colostrum-fed neonatal Holstein calves following intranasal vaccination with two commercially available modified-live virus vaccines. J Am Vet Med Assoc 2021;258:1119–29.

38. Tarabichi Y, Li K, Hu S, et al. The administration of intranasal live attenuated influ-enza vaccine induces changes in the nasal microbiota and nasal epithelium gene expression profiles. Microbiome 2015;3:74.

39. Mina MJ. Generalized herd effects and vaccine evaluation: impact of live influenza vaccine on off-target bacterial colonisation. J Infect 2017;74(Suppl 1): S101–7.

40. de Steenhuijsen Piters WAA, Jochems SP, Mitsi E, et al. Interaction between the nasal microbiota and S. pneumoniae in the context of live-attenuated influenza vaccine. Nat Commun 2019;10:2981.

41. Richeson JT, Beck PA, Gadberry MS, et al. Effects of on-arrival versus delayed modified live virus vaccination on health, performance, and serum infectious bovine rhinotracheitis titers of newly received beef calves. J Anim Sci 2008;86: 999–1005.

42. Richeson JT, Kegley EB, Gadberry MS, et al. Effects of on-arrival versus delayed clostridial or modified live respiratory vaccinations on health, performance, bovine viral diarrhea virus type I titers, and stress and immune measures of newly received beef calves. J Anim Sci 2009;87:2409–18.

43. Griffin CM, Scott JA, Karisch BB, et al. A randomized controlled trial to test the effect of on-arrival vaccination and deworming on stocker cattle health and growth performance. Bov Pract (Stillwater) 2018;52:26–33.

44. Snyder ER, Credille BC, Heins BD. Systematic review and meta-analysis comparing arrival versus delayed vaccination of high-risk beef cattle with 5-way modified-live viral vaccines against BHV-1, BRSV, PI3, and BVD types 1 and 2. Bovine Pract 2019;53:1–7.

45. Bosch AA, Biesbroek G, Trzcinski K, et al. Viral and bacterial interactions in the upper respiratory tract. PLoS Pathog 2013;9:e1003057.

46. McGillivary G, Mason KM, Jurcisek JA, et al. Respiratory syncytial virus-induced dysregulation of expression of a mucosal beta-defensin augments colonization of the upper airway by non-typeable Haemophilus influenzae. Cell Microbiol 2009; 11:1399–408.

47. Shilts MH, Rosas-Salazar C, Turi KN, et al. Nasopharyngeal Haemophilus and local immune response during infant respiratory syncytial virus infection. J Allergy Clin Immunol 2021;147:1097–101.e6.

48. de Steenhuijsen Piters WA, Heinonen S, Hasrat R, et al. Nasopharyngeal microbiota, host transcriptome, and disease severity in children with respiratory syncytial virus infection. Am J Respir Crit Care Med 2016;194:1104–15.

49. Zeineldin M, Lowe J, de Godoy M, et al. Disparity in the nasopharyngeal microbiota between healthy cattle on feed, at entry processing and with respiratory disease. Vet Microbiol 2017;208:30–7.

50. McMullen C, Alexander TW, Orsel K, et al. Progression of nasopharyngeal and tracheal bacterial microbiotas of feedlot cattle during development of bovine respiratory disease. Vet Microbiol 2020;248:108826.

51. Amat S, Timsit E, Baines D, et al. Development of bacterial therapeutics against the bovine respiratory pathogen Mannheimia haemolytica. Appl Environ Microbiol 2019;85.

52. Amat S, Alexander TW, Holman DB, et al. Intranasal bacterial therapeutics reduce colonization by the respiratory pathogen Mannheimia haemolytica in Dairy Calves. mSystems 2020;5:e00629.

53. Holman DB, Timsit E, Booker CW, et al. Injectable antimicrobials in commercial feedlot cattle and their effect on the nasopharyngeal microbiota and antimicrobial resistance. Vet Microbiol 2018;214:140–7.

54. Díaz-Pascual F, Hartmann R, Lempp M, et al. Breakdown of Vibrio cholerae biofilm architecture induced by antibiotics disrupts community barrier function. Nat Microbiol 2019;4:2136–45.

55. Snyder ER, Alvarez-Narvaez S, Credille BC. Genetic characterization of susceptible and multi-drug resistant *Mannheimia haemolytica* isolated from high-risk stocker calves prior to and after antimicrobial metaphylaxis. Vet Microbiol 2019; 235:110–7.
56. Crosby S, Credille B, Giguère S, et al. Comparative efficacy of enrofloxacin to that of tulathromycin for the control of bovine respiratory disease and prevalence of antimicrobial resistance in *Mannheimia haemolytica* in calves at high risk of developing bovine respiratory disease. J Anim Sci 2018;96:1259–67.
57. Holman DB, Yang W, Alexander TW. Antibiotic treatment in feedlot cattle: a longitudinal study of the effect of oxytetracycline and tulathromycin on the fecal and nasopharyngeal microbiota. Microbiome 2019;7:86.
58. Zeineldin M, Lowe J, Aldridge B. Effects of tilmicosin treatment on the nasopharyngeal microbiota of feedlot cattle with respiratory disease during the first week of clinical recovery. Front Vet Sci 2020;7:115.

Epidemiology's Adoption of System Dynamics is a Natural Extension of Population Thinking

David R. Smith, DVM, PhD[a],*, Robert W. Wills, DVM, PhD[b],
Kimberly A. Woodruff, DVM, MS[c]

KEYWORDS

- Epidemiology • BRD • Systems • Causal loop diagrams • Stock and flow models

KEY POINTS

- Epidemiologists use systems thinking to expand their understanding of the factors influencing the occurrence of health conditions beyond the linear relationships typically studied.
- Complex adaptive systems, such as beef cattle production systems, have a purpose and adjust to the conditions around them. Because they are complex, the response to surrounding conditions may not be predictable.
- Causal loop diagrams are graphical ways to communicate hypotheses about the relationships between various elements in a system, including feedback and time delays.
- Stock and flow models allow the quantification of various elements of a system and provide a means to test hypotheses developed through causal loop diagrams.
- Failing to understand the behavior of systems may lead to unintended or less than desirable outcomes.

INTRODUCTION

The discipline of epidemiology has been a recent adopter of systems thinking as a natural extension of the family of concepts of population medicine. Epidemiologists take a broad population-based perspective on understanding the health events that affect

[a] Department of Pathobiology and Population Medicine, Mississippi State University College of Veterinary Medicine, PO Box 6100, 240 Wise Center Drive, Mississippi State, MS 39762, USA;
[b] Department of Comparative Biomedical Sciences, Mississippi State University College of Veterinary Medicine, PO Box 6100, Mississippi State, MS 39762, USA; [c] Department of Clinical Sciences, Mississippi State University College of Veterinary Medicine, PO Box 6100, Mississippi State, MS 39762, USA
* Corresponding author.
E-mail address: dsmith@cvm.msstate.edu

Vet Clin Food Anim 38 (2022) 245–259
https://doi.org/10.1016/j.cvfa.2022.02.003
0749-0720/22/© 2022 Elsevier Inc. All rights reserved.
vetfood.theclinics.com

humans and animals. For example, health events might be a cow becoming pregnant, ground beef being contaminated with *Escherichia coli* O157:H7, or a neonatal calf developing diarrhea. Traditionally, epidemiologists have looked for relationships that explain the likelihood for these various health events. For example, by understanding the effect of low body condition on pregnancy rate, or that wet and muddy conditions increase the likelihood for feedlot steers to shed *E coli* O157:H7, whereas certain vaccines might reduce that risk, or that calves with failed transfer of passive immunity might be more likely to develop neonatal calf diarrhea. This approach to identifying causal risk factors has been useful for understanding why health events occur and it is hoped pointing to useful interventions. However, understanding these direct linear relationships between risk factor and event may not ensure long-term success in improving health outcomes. Even though commercialized vaccines were shown in several meta-analyses to reduce the risk for feedlot cattle to shed *E coli* O157:H7,[1,2,30] and models predicted that up to 85% of human illness from this foodborne pathogen might be prevented by vaccinating cattle,[3] virtually no cattle receive these vaccines. This is because the complex adaptive system of producing beef includes many players (eg, cow-calf producers, cattle feeders, beef processors, retailers, animal health industry, nutritionists, veterinarians, bankers, consumers, and regulators), often with competing interests and a lack of shared vision related to food safety. In total, the postharvest portion of the beef production system, most adversely affected by beef being contaminated with *E coli* O157:H7, could not find a way to reward the cattle feeder for administering the vaccine.[4] The science of systems thinking recognizes that underlying events and relationships lay a myriad of complex interactions that make up complex adaptive systems. Failing to understand the behavior of systems may lead to unintended or less than desirable outcomes.

BOVINE RESPIRATORY DISEASE AS AN EXAMPLE OF THINKING IN SYSTEMS

After 3 weeks of age, the leading cause of death of growing cattle, beef and dairy, is bovine respiratory disease (BRD).[5] Nearly 10% of beef calves in the United States may experience BRD before weaning[6] leading to the death of approximately 1% of beef calves while still with their dam.[7-9] Calves that recover from BRD in the preweaning period may weigh less at weaning compared with calves that were unaffected.[9,10]

Preweaning BRD occurs in 20% of beef cow-calf herds.[11,12] The annual cost to the cattle industry of BRD before weaning has been estimated to be $165 million because of death loss, treatment costs, and lost growth performance.[13] The labor to treat calves for BRD is variable depending on the production setting and may exceed the cost of medications.[14] The losses in the postweaning phase are much greater and BRD is the leading cause of sickness and death in beef finishing systems.[15,16] In the United States, BRD probably costs the postweaning phase of beef production $500 million per year.[16] Although BRD losses occur year-round, the fall and winter are the periods with the greatest death losses.[16]

Traditional Approaches to Bovine Respiratory Disease

The practitioner faced with an individual calf with BRD faces questions regarding how to treat the case. Their primary concerns are about whether antimicrobials are necessary, and if so, which antimicrobial to select for treatment, what dosage to use, and for what duration. They may wonder if ancillary therapy might help and consider the need for follow-up examination.

As we move from concern for the individual calf to concern for the population of calves, the practitioner may begin to wonder if the individual case should be managed in isolation from the rest of the herd and how to protect other calves in the herd from becoming ill. They may consider the value of control methods, such as vaccination in the face of an outbreak or metaphylactic antimicrobial therapy.

The traditional population-based approach to this scenario might be to try to understand the factors putting these calves at risk for BRD so that strategies are developed to prevent future outbreaks of disease or to know which biocontainment practices are most likely to reduce the number of new cases. Many factors contribute to the risk for BRD and epidemiologists have worked for many years to understand the direct linear relationship between various factors and the occurrence of BRD. For example, there are many viral and bacterial etiologic agents of BRD. Most BRD agents are endemic to cattle populations, but none are necessary or sufficient to cause disease.[17] Vaccines against these agents are commercially available and widely used in the United States. To be licensed, vaccine manufacturers must have demonstrated safety and efficacy in experimental studies. However, the efficacy of vaccines against preweaning BRD is weak or lacking when applied in beef production settings.[18,19] Even if the vaccines were effective, the logistics of timely immunization of calves against preweaning BRD in extensive cow-calf production settings are difficult. Having vaccines that reduced the risk for experimental infection has not been sufficient to prevent BRD in beef production systems.

SYSTEMS THINKING ABOUT BOVINE RESPIRATORY DISEASE

The overall incidence of BRD in the United States has not decreased, even though knowledge of the pathogens involved is better understood and the industry has the availability of better vaccines and antimicrobials.[16] One might wonder why the system of beef production would evolve to favor BRD pathogens. Epidemiologists have turned to systems thinking to help them better understand the decisions made by ranchers and cattle feeders that increase the likelihood of BRD in calves before and after weaning. System dynamics is a methodology that originated from the application of feedback control theory to the study of complex systems.[20] Through this approach, models that include not only cause and effect relationships, but also interactions, time delays, and feedback loops, are created to achieve a deeper understanding of the system. Simulation modeling using this nonlinear approach allows the modeler to observe the behavior of a system dynamically over time.[20,21] A system is a set of connected items that function together for a particular purpose. Complex adaptive systems, such as the beef production system, are dynamic systems able to adapt to and evolve with changes to external factors. Complex adaptive systems do not always behave the way one expects, and an important concern about modifying systems is creating unintended consequences.[21] Undesirable health outcomes in populations frequently result from not fully considering or understanding the system comprising the disease's ecology, including the decisions made by people responding to factors within the system (eg, biologic, or economic factors).

Biologic Systems

Compared with other domestic species, the anatomy and physiology of the bovine lung may make cattle inherently susceptible to BRD.[22] The occurrence of BRD in calves before weaning follows two distinct syndromes.[23] The first is a low incidence of BRD among calves less than 1 month of age, the other is a rapidly occurring outbreak of BRD among a large proportion of calves at a point in time when most calves in the herd are 3 to 5 months of age. These syndromes might be explained by failure of passive transfer of maternal antibodies in the case of the first syndrome, or the loss of herd immunity in the case of the second syndrome.[24] In the case of the latter, loss of herd immunity occurs after maternal immunity has waned in most calves in the herd. The half-life of maternally acquired IgG is 16 to 20 days, so by 5 half-lives (ie, when calves are 80–100 days of age) little maternal immunity remains to protect calves from systemic illnesses, such as BRD. In herds with short, seasonal calving seasons, many of the calves reach this state of reduced protection at about the same time, resulting in a sudden loss of herd immunity. Many calves have little or no antibodies against BRD pathogens at the time of marketing.[25,26] Also, the degree of internal parasitism at the time of arrival into a postweaning facility, as evidenced by eggs per gram in feces, is associated with increased risk for pneumonia. Unfortunately, deworming calves at arrival may not reduce morbidity or mortality, or improve growth performance.[26] Lower body weight of calves increases the risk for BRD.[17]

Production Systems

Producers may make management decisions that result in increased risk for BRD in their cattle, but those decisions do not necessarily reflect subpar husbandry, because they may be rational for other reasons. For example, preweaning BRD is a systems problem that is often, paradoxically, associated with highly managed herds.[11,12] Management practices, such as larger herd size, intensive grass management, and estrus synchronization, and shorter calving seasons are economically motivating to the cow-calf producer.[11] However, these same practices increase opportunities for effective contacts and transmission of BRD pathogens as calves lose herd immunity and the risk for preweaning BRD increases.

After beef calves are weaned, most are marketed from the cow-calf farm to an intermediate growing stage, variously known as stocker or backgrounding phases, or beef finishing feedlots. The average beef cow herd in the United States has just over 40 cows. Most beef cattle farms have less than 100 head of breeding females.[27] Many of the smaller cow-calf operations are part of a diversified farm system or provide supplemental income to off-farm employment.[27] Small cow-calf producers may lack the resources to prepare a calf to resist BRD pathogens after being marketed to the growing or finishing phases of beef production. For example, the farm may lack facilities, manpower, or knowledge to dehorn, castrate, deworm, or vaccinate calves before weaning. Calves from smaller herds with few facilities are often weaned on the same day they are transported to market, resulting in an abrupt stressful event. Beef calves are typically weaned at 6 to 8 months of age, coinciding with a decrease in available pasture forages, but that decision to wean and market calves unfortunately occurs at an age when calves have little immunity against BRD pathogens, which puts them at risk for postweaning BRD.[25,26]

Auction markets are vital for providing cow-calf producers, especially small farmers, an outlet to sell their calves in a transparent marketing system that allows for price discovery. Unfortunately, the auction marketing system may contribute additional stressors to calves. Calves may not know how to drink from water tanks or consume feed from bunks or they may not have access to adequate feed or water while transitioning through the market system. Although transitioning through the marketing system, calves are likely to be commingled with other calves, undergo long distance transportation, and they may spend several days in an order-buyer facility as other calves are purchased to fill an order. By the time calves arrive at the destination feedlot or stocker facility, they are likely to be exhausted, dehydrated, immunosuppressed by social and physical stressors, and incubating a respiratory pathogen.

It is a paradox that the marketing system may not reward the small cow-calf producer for adopting practices, such as early castration and dehorning, deworming, preweaning vaccination, or low-stress weaning methods, that might reduce the risk for BRD in the next phase of production. Commingled, low body condition, freshly weaned calves, transported long distances, and marketed through an auction market are often considered high risk for BRD. Yet interestingly, some cattle feeders and stocker operators prefer lightweight high-risk calves because they can be purchased for less total dollars and, if they survive, they may grow faster and more efficiently because of compensatory gains.[28] In contrast, the calves marketed from larger cow-calf ranches directly to the stocker or feedlot operation may experience few of the stressors of auction market calves. These calves are more likely to be better prepared to resist BRD pathogens because they have received deworming treatments, vaccination before weaning, and been castrated and dehorned at a young age because the value of calves marketed directly is often based on the rancher's reputation.

Most postweaning BRD occurs within 3 weeks of arrival into the growing or finishing facility. Feeding and finishing systems often attempt to reduce the probability for calves to develop BRD by vaccinating against BRD pathogens shortly after arrival, but vaccination at arrival may not reduce the incidence of BRD[18] and may sometimes increase BRD incidence, increase mortality, and reduce growth performance.[26] The most consistent method used by growing and finishing yards to reduce BRD incidence is mass medicating calves with injectable antimicrobials at arrival,[28] a practice that is receiving increased scrutiny because of concerns regarding antimicrobial resistance.

Altogether BRD is the outcome of a system that includes biologic components of the inherent susceptibility of the bovine lung, and a complex set of component causes including bacterial and viral pathogens, age-associated loss of immunity, environmental conditions that favor pathogen transmission, and stress-induced susceptibility. To these biologic factors are superimposed various production system decisions based on marketing, transportation, and economic opportunity that may further increase the risk for BRD at a critical age of susceptibility surrounding weaning age.

USING CAUSAL LOOP DIAGRAMS TO DESCRIBE SYSTEMS

Causal loop diagrams are useful tools for communicating hypotheses about how systems function, including feedback loops and time delays. Causal loop diagrams are a standardized graphical way to share hypotheses about systems more efficiently than by using the written or spoken word. The language starts with variables that are key components of the system. Variables are linked by arrows designating a causal relationship. Each arrow indicates whether the causal relationship is positive or negative (opposite or the same). The arrows are then designated with a positive or negative sign, or alternatively an "o" or "s," to indicate the relationship. Arrows also indicate how one variable might in turn have a feedback signal to the relationship. These feedback loops might be reinforcing or balancing. A reinforcing feedback loop continues to enhance the initiating factor. Balancing loops keep the initiating factor in check. Most systems have combinations of reinforcing and balancing loops and some pathways may be more dominant than others. Which pathways in the system dominates may depend on the strength of the feedback and delays that occur in sending signals.

A causal loop diagram illustrating the biologic and production system relationships that affect the risk for BRD in the postweaning phase is shown in **Fig. 1**. In this model the relationship between lightweight calves and profitability helps to explain why lightweight calves are economically desirable to cattle feeders, even though they have increased risk for developing BRD because of a variety of factors. The model also

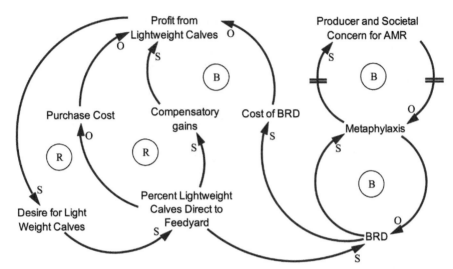

Fig. 1. A causal loop diagram to explain a hypothesized relationship between the occurrence of BRD and the number of lightweight calves directly entering finishing feedyards. In this model, profits from lower purchase price and increased growth performance (compensatory gains) of lightweight calves form reinforcing loops that continue to make lightweight calves desirable to cattle feeders. These relationships are balanced by the cost of BRD, which is more likely with lightweight calves. The incidence of BRD is balanced (mitigated) by metaphylactic use of antimicrobials at arrival, which makes the system continue to be profitable. Societal concern for antimicrobial resistance balances metaphylactic use (eg, by retail antimicrobial use policies). An *R in a circle* represents a reinforcing loop. A *B in a circle* represents a balancing loop. *Double hash marks* in an *arrow* indicate a time delay. AMR = antimicrobial resistance, BRD = bovine respiratory disease.

illustrates the role of metaphylactic use of antimicrobials to mitigate BRD costs to keep the system profitable. The selection for antimicrobial resistant bacteria may balance the practice of mass medicating calves with antimicrobials. Concern about antimicrobial resistance might affect the system through business and regulatory policies that discourage or forbid metaphylactic use of antimicrobials for BRD control. That change might then affect the value of lightweight calves to the cattle feeder which could fundamentally change the weaned calf market. Those market changes might affect how and where beef cattle are produced. By considering the relationships in the system of marketing and finishing beef calves, the epidemiologist may gain a better understanding of why BRD continues to plague the cattle industry despite better biologics and pharmaceuticals.

USING STOCK AND FLOW MODELS TO QUANTIFY PARAMETERS IN A SYSTEM

Stock and flow modeling (SFM) allows quantification of certain parameters of a system in a dynamic manner so that "what-if" scenarios can be run to test the effect of risk factors or the effectiveness of interventions. Construction of an SFM may provide a deeper understanding of the system's structure, identify knowledge gaps, and test the hypotheses generated through causal loop diagrams. The two most basic elements in an SFM are the stocks and the flows. A stock is an accumulation of a subject of interest. For example, stocks can be health outcomes, money, people, and so forth. Stocks are measured at points in time and, over time, accumulate through inflows and are depleted by outflows. In an SFM diagram, a stock is represented by a box.

Flows are control variables that influence the amount of stock. Flows, which are measured over time (time step), can increase, or decrease the amount of stock. In a diagram, flows are represented as valves. When flows originate outside of the system being studied, or outside of the model, they are represented in the model by a cloud shape.[21] A simple example of a stock and flow system is the amount of water in a bathtub. The amount of water, the element of interest, is the stock. The volume of water in the bathtub is increased by inflows (the faucet) or decreased by outflows (the drain).

STOCK AND FLOW MODEL OF A BOVINE RESPIRATORY DISEASE OUTBREAK

Previously, we discussed the practitioner's concern about what to do in the face of a BRD outbreak. An SFM might help to understand the nature of BRD outbreaks and perhaps how to mitigate them. For example, **Fig. 2** is an epidemic curve of new cases in an outbreak of BRD among 244 calves entering a feeding facility. These data were used to create an SFM, based on a Susceptible-Infected-Recovered model (**Fig. 3**) with the goal of producing an epidemic curve approximating the outbreak. The SFM was constructed using Vensim DSS 8.0.6 (Ventana Systems, Inc, Harvard, MA). Stocks in the model included Susceptible, Incubating, Infectious, and Recovered/Immune representing the number of calves in these different stages of disease dynamics. Calves transitioned from the Susceptible stock to the Incubating stock through the infecting flow, then to the Infectious stock through the transmission flow, and finally to the Recovered/Immune stock through the recovering flow. Modifiable parameters of the model included the Starting Population Size, Incubation Period, Initial Infectious, Contact Rate, Infectious Period, Probability of Infection, and Days at Order Buyer.

Susceptible Contacts were determined by multiplying the number of Susceptible calves by the Contact Rate. Total Population was calculated as the sum of the number of calves in all the stocks. The Proportion Infectious was the quotient of the number of

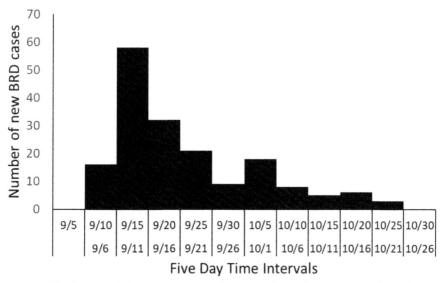

Fig. 2. Epidemic curve of bovine respiratory disease outbreak following arrival at a feedlot among 176 of 244 calves.

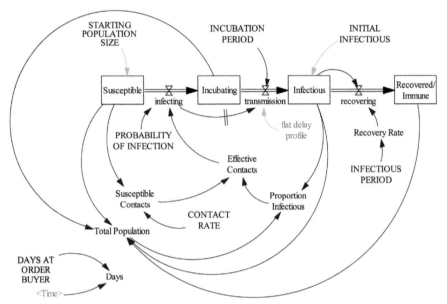

Fig. 3. Stock and flow model used to demonstrate the system dynamics of a bovine respiratory disease outbreak in calves in a feedlot.

Infectious calves divided by the Total Population. Susceptible Contacts was the product of the number of Susceptible calves and Contact Rate. In turn, the Effective Contacts was the product of Susceptible Contacts and Proportion Infectious. The rate of infecting was the product of Probability of Infection and Effective Contacts. The transition of calves from the Susceptible to the Infectious stocks was delayed in the Incubating stock by the effect of the Incubation Period on the transmission flow. The Recovery Rate, which was the reciprocal of the Infectious Period, determined the rate of the transition of calves from the Infectious stock to the Recovered/Immune stock by the recovering flow. The Days at Order Buyer allowed the calculation of the number of days before arrival of the calves in the feedlot that exposure to BRD pathogens could have occurred.

After the structure of the model was developed, modifiable parameters were initially populated with values that seemed appropriate through the experience of the authors and then adjusted until the SFM produced an epidemic curve, a plot of the number of calves in the Infectious stock over time (**Fig. 4**), which approximated the actual outbreak (**Fig. 2**). The number of calves in the Susceptible and Recovered/Immune stocks were also plotted to show the relationship of the three subpopulations of calves. Once this baseline SFM was established it was used to explore the system dynamics of the outbreak by changing individual parameters to see what effect they had on the levels of the Susceptible, Infectious, and Recovered/Immune stocks. The parameters used in the baseline SFM, and values used in scenarios with smaller or larger values, are listed in **Table 1**. It should be noted that the intent of this model is to demonstrate the utility of SFM to understand how dynamic behavior is affected by the structure of a system rather than professing to have identified the specific parameters of the modeled outbreak. In particular, the values chosen for the various scenarios were selected to demonstrate system dynamics rather than to model specific disease outbreaks.

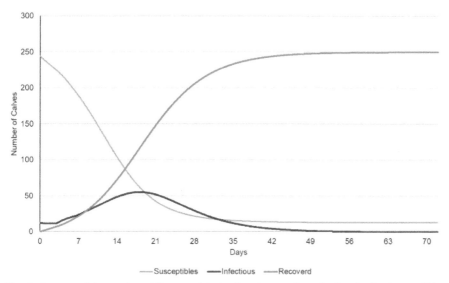

Fig. 4. Output of the stock and flow model plotting the number of calves in the Susceptible, Infectious, and Recovered stocks over time during an outbreak of bovine respiratory disease in a feedlot. The baseline parameters of the model were set at starting population size of 244 calves, 12 calves initially infected, incubation period of 3 days, infectious period of 5 days, contact rate of 12 calves per day, probability of infection of an effective contact of 0.05, and a 10-day period in the order buyer facility.

SCENARIOS

The baseline model was parameterized to approximate the BRD outbreak being used as an example. In **Fig. 4**, the levels in the Susceptibles stock decreased over time as calves became infected and transitioned into the Infectious stock while, simultaneously, calves recovering from disease moved from the Infectious stock to the Recovered/Immune stock. The peak number of infectious calves in the baseline model was 56 calves on Day 18 (see **Fig. 4**) compared with 58 calves on Day 9 (see **Fig. 2**) in the actual outbreak.

Table 1
Parameter values used for the baseline model and those used for scenarios in which a single parameter was decreased or increased from baseline levels to demonstrate how the model's stock values changed in response to the parameter changes

Parameters (Units)	Decreased Levels	Baseline Levels	Increased Levels
Starting population size of susceptibles (calves)	244	244	244
Contact rate (contacts/d)	6	12	18
Incubation period (d)	1	3	10
Infectious period (d)	1	5	9
Initially infectious (infectious calves)	2	12	22
Probability of infection	0.025	0.050	0.075
Days at order buyer barn (d)	10	10	10

Contact Rate

Decreasing the contact rate from 12 contacts/day to 6 contacts/day flattens the curve of the number of infectious calves (ie, epidemic curve) resulting in fewer susceptible calves becoming infectious and a corresponding delay in recovery of all animals when compared with the baseline scenario. Increasing the contact rate from 12 contacts/day to 18 contacts/day resulted in a higher and earlier peak number of infectious calves thereby depleting the number of susceptible calves earlier and more fully. These changes illustrate how reducing calf density and thereby potentially reducing contact rate can reduce the severity of an outbreak as is seen more clearly when plotting the epidemic curves for the three scenarios on one graph (**Fig. 5**).

Infectious Period

Decreasing the infectious period from baseline value of 5 days to 1 day dramatically decreases the magnitude of the outbreak with only a limited number of susceptible calves becoming infectious. Extending the infectious period to 9 days results in more rapid and sharper depletion of susceptible calves and increase in infectious calves. Effective use of antimicrobials might have a profound effect on the dynamics of a BRD outbreak by effectively altering the infectious period of infected calves (**Fig. 6**).

Number Initially Infectious

Reducing the number of calves that were initially infectious when brought to the feedlot from the baseline value of 12 infectious calves to 2 calves slowed the onset and rate of transition of susceptible to infectious calves. Increasing the number of calves initially infectious from baseline value of 12 calves to 22 calves resulted in a more rapid onset of the outbreak coupled with a higher peak number of infectious calves. The effect of the number of initially infectious calves on the onset of a BRD outbreak may explain the delayed clinical expression of the outbreak that sometimes

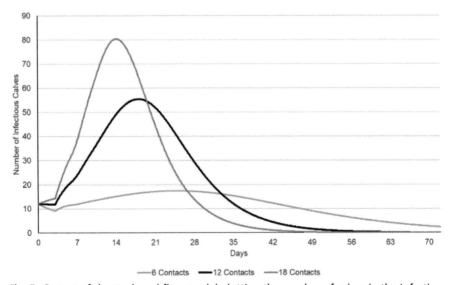

Fig. 5. Output of the stock and flow model plotting the number of calves in the Infectious stock over time (epidemic curves) during an outbreak of bovine respiratory disease in a feedlot with the contact rate set at 6, 12, or 18 contacts per day.

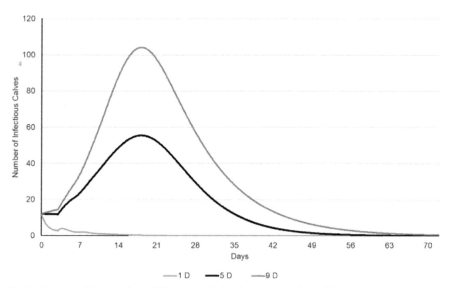

Fig. 6. Output of the stock and flow model plotting the number of infectious calves in over time (epidemic curves) during an outbreak of bovine respiratory disease in a feedlot with the infectious period set at 1, 5, or 9 days.

occurs among low-risk ranch direct cattle (**Fig. 7**).[29] Although not shown, the number of days spent at the order buyer facility before transportation to the feedlot may also affect the onset of clinical disease; longer times at the order buyer facility would allow more disease transmission within the facility and a higher number of infectious calves present on arrival resulting in a quicker onset of disease at the feedlot.

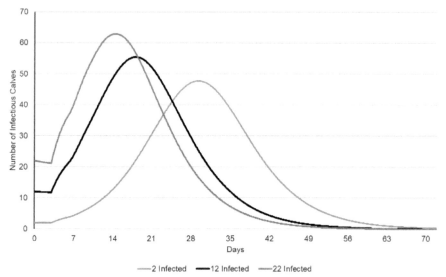

Fig. 7. Output of the stock and flow model plotting the number of calves in the Infectious stock over time (epidemic curves) during an outbreak of bovine respiratory disease in a feedlot with the initially infected calves set at 2, 12, or 22 calves.

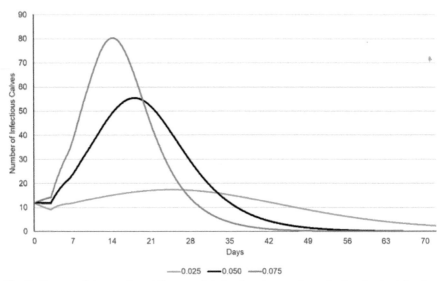

Fig. 8. Output of the stock and flow model plotting the number of calves in the Infectious stock over time (epidemic curves) during an outbreak of bovine respiratory disease in a feedlot with the probability of an effective contact becoming infected set at 0.025, 0.050, or 0.075.

Probability of Infection

Making changes to the probability of infection (**Fig. 8**) has an effect similar to changes in contact rate on the system dynamics of an outbreak because both parameters affect the rate of the infecting flow. The contact rate when multiplied by the number of susceptible calves determines the number of susceptible contacts. In turn, the number of effective contacts is calculated by multiplying the number of susceptible contacts by the proportion of infectious calves. The number of effective contacts multiplied by the probability of infection determines rate of the infecting flow. Proportional changes in either probability of infection or in contact rate result in the same change in the rate of the infecting flow. The probability of infection could be reduced by use of antimicrobials to decrease the probability of infection when an effective contact is created.

In summary, the SFM is useful to have a general understanding of the system dynamics of an outbreak of BRD or other diseases. Although not done for this demonstration model, an SFM could be created that closely adheres to the structure and parameters of a specific disease and feedlot system so that outcomes that more precisely reflect changes occurring in response to interventions could be assessed. However, it is often not necessary for an SFM to closely model reality to be useful.

SUMMARY

Epidemiologists have adopted systems thinking as an approach to better understand the complex interactions of factors that lead to undesirable health events. Causal loop diagrams and SFM help to better understand the complex dynamic nature of beef production systems and the effect of decisions, sometimes made long before or far away, on health outcomes.

ACKNOWLEDGMENTS

A contribution of the Beef Cattle Population Health and Reproduction Program at Mississippi State University. Supported by the Mikell and Mary Cheek Hall Davis Endowment for Beef Cattle Health and Reproduction and the Agriculture and Food Research Initiative Competitive Grants Program Grant no. 2018 69003 28706 from the USDA National Institute of Food and Agriculture. Any opinions, finding, conclusions, or recommendations expressed in this article are those of the authors and do not necessarily reflect the view of the US Department of Agriculture.

CLINICS CARE POINTS

- causal loop diagrams help to communicate our thoughts about how the components of a system interact.
- Stock and flow models help us quantify system behaviors.
- Some system modelers prefer to develop causal loop diagrams before creating the stock and flow model. Others prefer to create the stock and flow model first and let those results inform the causal loop diagram.

DISCLOSURE

The authors have no conflicts of interest to disclose.

REFERENCES

1. Snedeker KG, Campbell M, Sargeant JM. A systematic review of vaccinations to reduce the shedding of *Escherichia coli* O157 in the faeces of domestic ruminants. Zoonoses Public Health 2012;59:126–38.
2. Vogstad AR, Moxley RA, Erickson GE, Klopfenstein TJ, Smith DR. Stochastic Simulation Model Comparing Distributions of STEC O157 Faecal Shedding Prevalence Between Cattle Vaccinated With Type III Secreted Protein Vaccines and Non-Vaccinated Cattle. Zoonoses Public Health 2014;61:283–9.
3. Matthews L, Reeve R, Gally DL, et al. Predicting the public health benefit of vaccinating cattle against *Escherichia coli* O157. Proc Natl Acad Sci U S A 2013;110: 16265–70.
4. Smith DR, Vogstad AR. Vaccination as a method of *E. coli* O157:H7 reduction in feedlot cattle. In: Callaway TR, Edrington TS, editors. On farm strategies to control foodborne pathogens. Hauppauge, NY: Nova Science Publishers Inc.; 2012.
5. USDA. Cattle Death Loss. Washington, DC: U.S. Dept. of Agriculture ASB, National Agricultural Statistics Service; 2011.
6. Hanzlicek GA, Renter DR, White BJ, et al. Management practices associated with the rate of respiratory tract disease among preweaned beef calves in cow-calf operations in the United States. J Am Vet Med Assoc 2013;242:1271–8.
7. USDA. Beef 2007–08, Part IV: reference of beef cow-calf management practices in the United States, 2007–08. Fort Collins, CO: USDA:APHIS:VS, CEAH; 2010. #523.0210.
8. Dutil L, Fecteau G, Bouchard E, et al. A questionnaire on the health, management, and performance of cow-calf herds in Quebec. Can Vet J 1999;40:649–56.

9. Snowder GD, Van Vleck LD, Cundiff LV, et al. Influence of breed, heterozygosity, and disease incidence on estimates of variance components of respiratory disease in preweaned beef calves. J Anim Sci 2005;83:1247–61.

10. Wittum TE, Salman MD, King ME, et al. The influence of neonatal health on weaning weight of Colorado, USA beef calves. Prev Vet Med 1994;19:15–25.

11. Woolums AR, Berghaus RD, Smith DR, et al. Producer survey of herd-level risk factors for nursing beef calf respiratory disease. J Am Vet Med Assoc 2013; 243:538–47.

12. Woolums AR, Berghaus RD, Smith DR, et al. A survey of veterinarians in 6 US states regarding their experience with nursing beef calf respiratory disease. Bovine Pract 2014;48:9.

13. Wang M, Schneider LG, Hubbard KJ, et al. Cost of bovine respiratory disease in preweaned calves on US beef cow-calf operations (2011-2015). J Am Vet Med Assoc 2018;253:624–31.

14. Wang M, Schneider LG, Hubbard KJ, et al. Beef producer survey of the cost to prevent and treat bovine respiratory disease in preweaned calves. J Am Vet Med Assoc 2018;253:617–23.

15. Griffin D. Feedlot diseases. Vet Clin North Am Food Anim Pract 1998;14:199–231.

16. Miles DG. Overview of the North American beef cattle industry and the incidence of bovine respiratory disease (BRD). Anim Health Res Rev 2009;10:101–3.

17. Taylor JD, Fulton RW, Lehenbauer TW, et al. The epidemiology of bovine respiratory disease: what is the evidence for predisposing factors? Can Vet J 2010;51: 1095–102.

18. Taylor JD, Fulton RW, Lehenbauer TW, et al. The epidemiology of bovine respiratory disease: what is the evidence for preventive measures? Can Vet J 2010;51: 1351–9.

19. Larson RL, Step DL. Evidence-based effectiveness of vaccination against *Mannheimia haemolytica*, *Pasteurella multocida*, and *Histophilus somni* in feedlot cattle for mitigating the incidence and effect of bovine respiratory disease complex. Vet Clin North Am Food Anim Pract 2012;28:97–106, 106e101-107, ix.

20. Forrester JW. Industrial dynamics. Cambridge (MA): M.I.T. Press; 1961.

21. Meadows DH, Wright D. Thinking in systems: a primer. White River Junction (VT): Chelsea Green Pub.; 2008. p. 23.

22. Veit HP, Farrell RL. The anatomy and physiology of the bovine respiratory system relating to pulmonary disease. Cornell Vet 1978;68:555–81.

23. Smith DR. Field epidemiology to manage BRD risk in beef cattle production systems. Anim Health Res Rev 2014;15(2):180–3.

24. Smith DR. Management to decrease neonatal calf loss in beef herds. In: Hopper R, editor. Bovine reproduction. 2nd ed. Hoboken, NJ: John Wiley and Sons; 2021. p. 899–908.

25. Step DL, Krehbiel CR, Burciaga-Robles LO, et al. Comparison of single vaccination versus revaccination with a modified-live virus vaccine containing bovine herpesvirus-1, bovine viral diarrhea virus (types 1a and 2a), parainfluenza type 3 virus, and bovine respiratory syncytial virus in the prevention of bovine respiratory disease in cattle. J Am Vet Med Assoc 2009;235:580–7.

26. Griffin CM, Scott JA, Karisch BB, et al. A randomized controlled trial to test the effect of on-arrival vaccination and deworming on stocker cattle health and growth performance. Bov Pract (Stillwater) 2018;52:26–33.

27. Davis CG. Cattle and beef. Sector at a glance. Washington, DC: U.S. Dept. of Agriculture ERS; 2021.

28. Ives SE, Richeson JT. Use of antimicrobial metaphylaxis for the control of bovine respiratory disease in high-risk cattle. Vet Clin North Am Food Anim Pract 2015; 31:341–50, v.
29. Theurer ME, Johnson MD, Fox T, et al. Bovine respiratory disease during the mid-portion of the feeding period: observations from vaccination history, viral and bacterial prevalence, and rate of gain in feedlot cattle. Appl Anim Sci 2021;37: 59–67.
30. Varela NP, Dick P, Wilson J. Assessing the existing information on the efficacy of bovine vaccination against Escherichia coli O157:H7–a systematic review and meta-analysis. Zoonoses Public Health 2013;60:253–68.

The Sandhills Calving System—Putting Systems Thinking into Practice

Halden Clark, DVM, MS

KEYWORDS

- Sandhills • Calving • Neonatal calf diarrhea • Systems thinking

KEY POINTS

- Intensification of management within beef herds over time may have led to risk factors increasing the likelihood for neonatal calf diarrhea outbreaks in the production system.
- These risk factors include early calving seasons, long calving seasons, calving heifers and cows on wintering grounds, calving heifers and cows together, increasing group size, and others.
- Although treatment has efficacy, veterinarians and producers were unable to curtail losses to this disease by symptomatic treatment alone.
- Treatment incentivized concentration of animals, which exacerbated the disease outbreak. This is an example of a vicious cycle, or "reinforcing feedback loop" in the terminology of the discipline of Systems Thinking.
- The Sandhills Calving System has been shown to reduce the incidence of neonatal calf diarrhea in beef herds and is an example of a system modification at a point of leverage that has demonstrated positive downstream effects.
- The Sandhills Calving System may serve as a helpful example of several Systems Thinking concepts.

INTRODUCTION

Beef cattle production exists as a complex adaptive system. Factors such as cattle and feed prices, labor availability, interest rates, and land values are constantly changing, and place pressures on beef cattle producers to move toward production intensification. In commodity markets over time, price is equal to [average] cost of production.[1] Herd owners and managers must adapt to rapidly changing economic forces to stay competitive within the challenging commodity marketplace. Often, changes that are made to stay competitive in beef production can have unforeseen animal health implications. Among the changes adopted by cattle producers to

University of Nebraska-Lincoln, Great Plains Veterinary Educational Center, Clay Center, PO Box 148, 820 Road 313, NE 68933, USA
E-mail address: hclark16@unl.edu

Vet Clin Food Anim 38 (2022) 261–271
https://doi.org/10.1016/j.cvfa.2022.03.003
0749-0720/22/© 2022 Elsevier Inc. All rights reserved.
vetfood.theclinics.com

improve production efficiency and economic returns are genetic selection to increase individual animal productivity, increases in herd size, reduction in labor requirements per animal, and timing calving season to optimize calf marketing opportunities. Many cow/calf operations concentrated herds in corrals and close to windbreaks that provided protection from adverse weather events while also allowing easy access to calving facilities and equipment. Aspects of these changes may have led to the accumulation of risk factors for outbreaks of neonatal calf diarrhea. This situation can serve as an example of a Systems Thinking concept called "Limits to Success," which suggests that as attempts are made to optimize a system, such as beef production in temperate climates, unforeseen barriers may arise that limit the ability of the system to grow unimpeded. The Sandhills Calving System (SCS) is an example of a system modification at a point of leverage that addresses the root causes of this "limit to success" (neonatal calf diarrhea) and controls them while still allowing many of the benefits of beef production intensification to be captured.

Fig. 1 shows a "causal loop diagram," which is an effort to explore and connect causes that may have led to observed downstream phenomena.

CHANGES WITHIN BEEF HERDS BEFORE THE DEVELOPMENT OF THE SANDHILLS CALVING SYSTEM
Genetic Changes Within the National Beef Herd

Beef production intensification efforts included genetic selection for larger and increasingly heavily muscled and high growth-rate beef animals.[2] Later efforts brought in double-muscled cattle with 1 or 2 nonfunctional myostatin alleles,[3] lines of cattle selected to have dizygotic twin calves,[4] and more. Many of these pursuits were associated with increased risk of dystocia as well,[3,4] which would incentivize concentrating

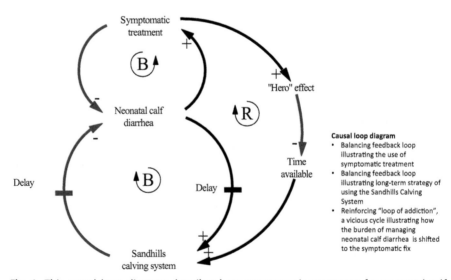

Fig. 1. This causal loop diagram describes how symptomatic treatment for neonatal calf diarrhea may alleviate the problem in the short term but may absorb the time resources needed to address it at a more fundamental level through Sandhills Calving System methods.

animals near handling facilities around the time of calving season to be able to address dystocia cases. Historically, cattle dystocia rates were presumably low in the United States in the Civil War era and afterward as feral cattle and Longhorns underwent selection pressure against dystocia due to lack of active animal husbandry.[2] Later, as some of these cattle were crossed with and eventually largely replaced by British and Continental European beef breeds,[2] dystocia rates appear to have climbed across the industry. The intensification efforts described earlier were likely a part of this.

Dystocia appears to have been a very significant problem within beef production immediately before the development of the SCS. A 1994 review article by Dr Lawrence Rice noted that at that time, 64% of calf losses between birth and weaning were due to dystocia.[5] Although not US-based, the author cites European Economic Community data showing that between 1.8% and 9.4% of all beef calves died due to dystocia at that time. Twenty-three years later, the National Animal Health Monitoring Service (NAHMS) 2017 survey suggests much lower dystocia rates. In this survey, producers reported that across all regions and herd sizes in the United States, calf death losses from all causes before weaning were between 2.8% and 3.8%, averaging 3.3%. Of these, no more than 24.7% of those losses were due to dystocia, and possibly significantly less due to unclear total losses distributed between age groups of less than 3 weeks of age versus 3 weeks of age to weaning. This would translate into losses to dystocia of no greater than 0.8% of all calves born. In addition, these producers indicated that respiratory disease, predators, and unknown causes each outranked dystocia as causes of death in 2017 in calves between calving and weaning.

In 1992 to 1993, NAHMS' Cow/Calf Health and Productivity Audit (CHAPA) recorded that in heifers, 11% of all calvings were classified by producers as a "hard pull." This same number was 5.1% in 1997, 3.4% in 2007 to 2008, and 3.0% in 2017.

In 1992 to 1993, 1.2% of heifers are reported as needing Caesarean-section surgeries to deliver calves. In 2017, only 0.2% of heifers are reported as needing Caesarean sections according to CHAPA and NAHMS data.

As the previous information suggests, dystocia rates appear to have declined over the last 20 to 25 years. Utilization of bulls that were selected to promote calving ease likely played an important role in this.[6] An in-depth exploration of each of these factors is beyond the scope of this article, but the pressure toward intensification appears to have driven dystocia rates up, until efforts were made to reduce them through changes to bull selection and heifer development.

The author's personal communications with practitioners in Nebraska indicate that in some areas in the 1990s, individual beef veterinarians commonly performed an average of 200 or more Caesarean-section surgeries annually, and in the same areas, average annual Caesarean sections had gradually fallen to less than 20 per veterinarian recently. Cow numbers in those areas had declined over that time as well, but marginally.

In the years before the development of the SCS, dystocia may have provided an incentive for cattle managers to concentrate cattle near handling facilities during calving season to be better able to observe periparturient females and render assistance during difficult calvings in a timely fashion. This concentration of animals would have likely led to the introduction of neonatal calf diarrhea risk factors. These factors are linked in the causal loop diagram shown in **Fig. 1**.

Herd Size Changes

The United States Department of Agriculture's National Agriculture Statistics Service records Census of Agriculture data that include a variety of beef cattle statistics, and the most recent took place in 2017. Though since 1992, the nationwide average herd size has only gone from 37 cows per herd to 43.5 cows per herd in 2017, individual herds may have grown to a much greater extent as numerous small herds are likely kept for nonmonetary reasons, as the NAHMS 2011 Small-scale US Cow-calf Operations Report shows. In 2017, all sizes of beef operations over 50 head reported growth in the total numbers of operations in existence of 7% to 13% from the prior Census of Agriculture in 2012. Operations with more than 1000 cows increased by 8%. In 2017, 54% of beef cows in the United States were in herds with more than 100 head. For comparison, in Nebraska, the average cow/calf herd size was 69 cows in 1987, and 107 cows by 2017.

Herd size has been identified as an independent risk factor for neonatal calf diarrhea[7] but may also act as an indirect risk factor by further incentivizing concentration of animals to efficiently use labor. It has been documented that death losses in calves are greater when employees provide animal care than when cattle owners provide care.[8] Possible reasons for this may include the owner often having greater freedom to implement preventive care and to limit stressors and other risk factors for animal disease than employees. As herd sizes increase, the likelihood that animal caretakers are employees rather than owners increases as well. These inter-relationships are also represented in the causal loop diagram shown in **Fig. 1**.

Risk Factors for Neonatal Calf Diarrhea

A 1994 review article lays out the risk factors known at the time regarding neonatal calf diarrhea.[9] The author of that article calculates that a beef veterinary practice should expect that approximately 4% to 16% of their producers would experience what he terms unacceptably high calf mortality due to neonatal calf diarrhea each year at the time the article was written. This suggests that at the time, neonatal calf diarrhea was a widespread and costly problem. He goes on to describe the shift from a typical April/May calving window back toward January 1st that was significantly affecting the industry when the article was written. This change was occurring to capitalize on October and November prices for heavier calves.

Earlier calving season with poorly drained ground in the nursing areas have been associated with higher risk of neonatal calf diarrhea.[7,10] With earlier calving season comes a higher likelihood that cows will calve in barns and sheds, and these are a risk factor for neonatal calf diarrhea when space per animal is limited.[10] The review article cites unpublished data that showed that calves born in pens with 1000 square feet of pen space per cow-calf pair were at lower risk of calf diarrhea than were calves born in pens with 250 square feet of pen space per cow-calf pair.[9] Other studies indicate an increased risk of calf diarrhea in calves born to heifers, herds that calve heifers and cows together, and high stocking densities.[7,10,11] Risk of high calf mortality went up with longer calving season duration and with larger herds.[7,10-12] NAHMS data from 2007 show that 23.2% of beef producers with herds 1 to 49 head agreed or strongly agreed that neonatal calf diarrhea had a significant economic impact on their operations, compared with 45.4% of those with herds from 50 to 99 head, 54.3% of those with herds 100 to 199 head, and 57.6% of those with herds 200 head or more. Veterinarians at that time (before introduction of the SCS) recommended a list of preventive interventions centered around reduced stocking density, limiting group size to 50 head if possible, calving onto pen surfaces with minimal contamination, and separating heifers from cows.[13] These recommendations show that at the time, veterinarians had a substantial knowledge of the risk factors for neonatal calf scours but did not appear to have yet identified an important point of leverage in preventing the disease that would later be used in the SCS, which was breaking the chain of pathogen transmission from older to younger calves.

Treatment of Sick Calves

In the middle of a neonatal calf diarrhea outbreak, cattle owners or managers responsible for treating sick calves could have been further incentivized to confine the herd closer to the available cattle working facilities to improve efficiency in getting calves caught and treated (author's personal communications with practitioners in NE and MO). This could lead to increasing pathogen load in the calving environment and likely a worsening of the incidence rate and severity of neonatal calf diarrhea. This is an example of vicious cycle, also called in Systems Thinking terminology a reinforcing feedback loop (**Fig. 2**) in which efforts to treat the disease may have led to perpetuating or even worsening of the outbreak.

Vaccination as Prevention

Early efforts to prevent the disease may likewise have met with difficulty. Vaccination can be an ideal intervention against infectious disease in beef herds in some cases. Many vaccinations cost less than the price of feed for a cow for several days, and if effective, may reduce the need for expensive infrastructure upgrades. In addition, if no system-level changes are necessary to prevent the disease, the burden on the cattle manager to predict downstream consequences of the intervention is reduced. Because of these considerations, vaccination may often appear highly desirable as a possible intervention for beef cattle disease prevention.

It is necessary, however, for the vaccinations in question to be efficacious for this to be a functional solution. An overview of the extensive research into individual neonatal calf diarrhea pathogens and the numerous commercial vaccines available against them is beyond the scope of this article. Although the various vaccines designed to prevent neonatal calf diarrhea may have shown efficacy in challenge models, there are few field studies in the literature. Field studies that exist have equivocal findings,[14] lack features like blinding, randomization, and commingling information,[15] or are from overseas in substantially different production systems.[16] Thus, the veterinary practitioner is left with a scarcity of evidence of field efficacy to support usage decisions. In addition, other studies have shown that herds that vaccinate for neonatal calf diarrhea are at higher risk of the disease than herds that do not.[7] The reason for this is

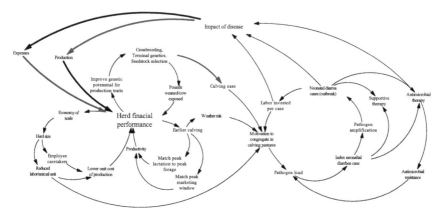

Fig. 2. Causal loop diagram: describes theorized relationships between factors within a complex system. Blue lines: contributes to or increases downstream factor. Red lines: decreases downstream factor.

unknown but may be that those herds carry more risk factors and overwhelm the immunity provided by the vaccines. If vaccine use were attempted without addressing pathogen amplification or pathogen load, the results may have been unsatisfying.[17]

Rotational Grazing as Prevention

Rotational grazing methods alone did not appear to prevent neonatal calf diarrhea outbreaks from occurring despite frequent moves to uncontaminated pastures.[18,19] This suggests that pathogens loads can develop quickly when calf-to-calf transmission is not prevented.

FINDING A POINT OF LEVERAGE

It appears that incentives for cattle owners and managers to concentrate cattle near handling facilities may have converged in the 1990s, just before when the SCS was developed. Factors involved included higher dystocia rates, larger herds, reduced labor per cow, and the need to treat calves with neonatal calf diarrhea. This hypothesis is represented by the causal loop diagram. If accurate, these factors, which can be viewed as the results of intensification efforts, may have set up conditions for neonatal calf diarrhea to fall into what is termed a "vicious reinforcing feedback loop." This would allow neonatal calf diarrhea losses to essentially worsen over time, and act as a limit to intensification successes.

The SCS appears to provide an exit from the reinforcing feedback loop discussed earlier. The following explanation of the development of the SCS is a retrospective attempt to elucidate how veterinarians' efforts may serve as an example of the process of thinking through a system and designing an intervention. The following information was gathered through personal communication between several of the original developers of the SCS and the author.

The development of the SCS began in the early 1990s, when the incentives to concentrate cattle described earlier may have been strong. The risk factors had largely been identified, and prevention through vaccination and some calving season management methods had been attempted and may have met with some success. However, at that time, several herds struggling with severe yearly neonatal calf diarrhea outbreaks during and after calving season sought help from veterinarians, ruminant nutritionists, and University extension personnel in Nebraska. Interdisciplinary teams were formed that met at ranches to search for ways to learn about the problems being encountered. Each was able to explain perspectives and experiences with neonatal calf diarrhea outbreaks. A process of careful reasoning is a hallmark of efforts to work toward a better understanding of a complex system.

Epidemiologic Methods Were Applied

Veterinary researchers began applying epidemiologic techniques to the neonatal calf diarrhea problem on several ranches that were struggling with outbreaks. By creating epidemic curves and looking at risk of disease and death by date born (**Fig. 3**), the team realized that the outbreak frequently started 3 to 4 weeks after calving season began, and risk of disease and death from neonatal calf diarrhea increased rapidly in calves born later in the calving season.[19] Consistently, the latest-born calves were at many times higher risk of death than the calves born at the beginning of calving season. Area veterinarians and ranchers confirmed that this fit the clinical picture that they were familiar with, and the findings were similar from ranch to ranch. Careful observers with differing perspectives began to integrate their viewpoints, and a better understanding of the phenomenon was achieved.

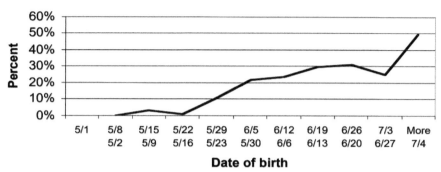

Fig. 3. The proportion of calves born each week that subsequently died due to neonatal calf diarrhea. Calves born later in the calving season had increasingly greater risk of death. Data are from Case Herd #2 before implementing the Sandhills Calving System. (*From* Smith DR, Grotelueschen DM, Knott T, Clowser SL, Nason G. Population Dynamics of Undifferentiated Neonatal Calf Diarrhea among Ranch Beef Calves. Bov Pract 2008, 42:1, page 5, with permission.)

Examining the available literature revealed that fecal samples from herds with numerous calves less than 2 months of age, high stocking densities, and long calving seasons were more likely to be shedding *Cryptosporidium parvum* oocysts.[18] This led to the suspicion that a "multiplier effect" may exist in calves that caused pathogen amplification in the calving pen or pasture. It was further posited that this may involve more of the commonly implicated pathogens than *Cryptosporidium* alone, since the clinical picture was similar, though not identical, across the various calf diarrhea pathogens. The team hypothesized that the buildup of pathogenic bacteria, viruses, and protozoa in the immediate calving environment and the shedding of pathogens from older calves to younger calves were significant factors contributing to the high rates of mortality in the latest-born calves. This idea was supported indirectly by outbreak data showing that calves born in the later weeks of calving season are at much higher risk of dying from neonatal calf diarrhea than calves born at the beginning of calving season.[19] It appeared that the first few calves in the sequence may not show symptoms of disease, but calves later in the sequence may receive higher infective doses of pathogens and could show symptoms, sicken, and in some cases die. Biocontainment of pathogens already found within the cattle populations on each operation was identified as the point of leverage at which an intervention might be most powerful. Specifically, the age-segregation of neonatal calves from calves several weeks older, which may be shedding large volumes of one or more of the known calf diarrhea pathogens, was that point of leverage.[20]

Hypotheses Were Tested in On-Farm, Applied Research Trials

In a 2003 Range Beef Cow Symposium presentation, researchers shared data from 2 ranches. In the 3 to 5 years before implementing the SCS, the 2 ranches had been struggling with neonatal calf diarrhea death losses ranging from 6% to 15% of calf crop year after year. It had caused significant emotional stress, workload, medical expense, and financial losses on both operations. Both ranches decided to implement the SCS and mapped out when and how they would make the necessary pasture moves well ahead of calving season. The first ranch had between 800 and 900 cows, and the second had 400. After implementing the SCS, and until the end of a 3-year follow-up, neither of the ranches that implemented Sandhills Calving methods lost a single calf to neonatal calf diarrhea, and never treated more than 3.[21]

Clinics Care Points: the Core of the Sandhills Calving System

The SCS is typically implemented in the following way.[20]

- For the first 1-2 weeks of calving season, the entire cow herd is together in the first pen or pasture.
- After calving has gone on for 1-2 weeks there, all the still-pregnant "heavy" cows are moved to the second calving pasture.
- The pairs from the first 1-2 weeks of calving remain in the first calving pasture.
- After another week, all the cows that have yet to calve are again moved to the third pasture, and the calves born on pasture 2 stay there with their dams.
- After another week, all the heavy cows are moved ahead to the fourth pasture, and so on, until calving season is over.
- When the youngest calves are at least 1 month old, the groups are reassembled.

The schematic in **Fig. 4** provides a snapshot of the SCS at week 5 of calving season. This method allows calves to be born onto fresh pastures and remain with their 7-day "age cohorts" of calves through their first month of life. It prevents 1- to 4-week-old calves, which may be shedding large volumes of viral, bacterial, and protozoal pathogens, from inundating the newborn calves with heavy infectious doses. When the youngest calves are one month old, groups of calves have been reassembled without precipitating a subsequent neonatal calf diarrhea outbreak. Planning pen or pasture usage according to this methodology attempts to recreate conditions present at the beginning of calving season in subsequent moves of pregnant animals to a relatively uncontaminated environment. Age-segregation of calves attempts to interrupt the chain of transmission of heavy loads of calf diarrhea pathogens from older calves to neonatal calves.[20]

Week 5

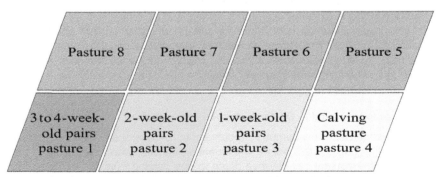

Fig. 4. Schematic of the Sandhills Calving System in the fifth week of calving season. During week 5, cows are calving in the fourth pasture and calves born in the previous pastures remain behind in similar-age groups. (*Courtesy of* Dr. David R. Smith, Starkville, MS)

Utilization of SCS

Because the SCS involves initiating the calving season with several pens or pastures that have not had cattle in them for at least several months, there is often a significant time investment in planning. Effective planning often helps to better use existing facilities, but it is possible that additional infrastructure (fencing, etc) may be required as well. This process often works best if initiated well ahead of time, often many months before the onset of calving. Perhaps even more paramount in preparations for the adoption of the SCS is addressing the current mental models (**Box 1**) that exist as part of the operational culture of the ranch regarding calving pasture management. Knowledge regarding calving pasture management is often acquired through experience and through the intergenerational training that is ingrained into the ranching enterprise. Asking individuals to examine such deeply held mental models requires intimate working relationships between veterinarians and producers.

"Shifting the Burden" Archetype

It appears that for the ranches on which the SCS was initially implemented, simply focusing on treatment alone for neonatal calf diarrhea without looking for methods of prevention would serve as an example of a "Shifting the Burden" archetype in Systems Thinking terminology.[22] A Shifting the Burden archetype could be described as follows. Focusing on sick calf treatment can be seen as a "symptomatic" fix that only addresses the symptoms of deeper problems. It yields quick results, but underlying causes are unaddressed. Focusing on age cohort biocontainment using the SCS can be seen at the fundamental root cause fix. This takes planning and long-term effort, as discussed earlier. Focusing more effort on the symptomatic fix (working harder to treat more diarrheic calves) undermines the ability to redirect resources to the fundamental fix, which is biocontainment throughout calving season. An additional aspect of a Shifting the Burden situation is termed the "Hero Effect." This suggests that when short term, symptomatic fixes are successful, there is either intrinsic (eg, person is happy calf survived) or extrinsic (eg, person receives bonus pay) positive reinforcement given to the person who applied the treatment. Beyond just taking up time that might otherwise be spent addressing root causes, this effect also actively incentivizes the person to continue applying treatment to the symptoms as doing so yields immediate rewards, potentially further reducing the person's motivation to pursue the fundamental fix.

In herds with numerous risk factors and significant outbreaks, vaccination may also replace symptomatic treatment in a "Shifting the Burden" diagram. This could occur if

---

Box 1
Mental Models

- They can be conscious or unconscious.

- They are critical to our effectiveness.

- They affect how we think and how we act.

- It is easier to see others' mental models than to see our own.

- They are always incomplete and often flawed.

- They are high leverage.

adding a vaccination in a production system that consistently develops a heavy pathogen load in the calving and nursing areas gives the cattle manager a sense that the problem has been fully addressed. If taking this action reduces the impetus needed to address root causes, animal health could suffer before fundamental fixes are pursued.

Sandhills Calving Illustrates the Potential of Modifying a System at a Point of Leverage

The SCS is an example of the potential for thinking in systems and illustrates how deepening our understanding of a beef operation's entire system can lead to remarkable successes for those who are willing to consider a structural change and to go through the process of planning and implementing it. In the years since, there has been significant uptake of these ideas by beef producers. National Animal Health Monitoring Service (NAHMS) data from 2017 show that 27% of cow/calf operations of all sizes use some form of Sandhills Calving in the central region (NE, KS, SD, ND, MN, IA, MO). It also shows that 40% of beef cow/calf operations across the United States that have more than 200 cows use the main principles of Sandhills Calving. Clearly, if farms continue to struggle with neonatal calf diarrhea outbreaks while not using SCS principles, there is still room for growth. However, for a system less than 25 years old, this appears to be considerable industry uptake.

DISCUSSION

Changes in beef cow/calf herd management may have led to the need for the SCS, but further changes also aided the SCS. Lower dystocia rates since the development of the SCS likely helped reduce the need for concentrating heifers and cows near calving facilities. Design and sales of portable panels and calving stalls may have made addressing dystocia on pastures more convenient. Perhaps in moderate-sized herds, the need for splitting cows and heifers into different calving units would add labor needs, but further herd growth on some ranches may have made calving heifers and cows separately less of a labor demand as both groups are large enough to require substantial labor investment on their own. As described earlier, the SCS may represent one of the clearest examples within beef veterinary medicine of a system modification at a point of leverage that led to positive downstream effects. These effects include reducing or eliminating calf illness and death loss due to neonatal calf diarrhea, improved economic performance of the beef operation, reductions in need for antimicrobial drug utilization, reductions in labor to treat sick calves, reductions in human emotional stress and zoonotic disease risk, and improved animal welfare.

DISCLOSURE

The author has nothing to disclose.

REFERENCES

1. Maddux J. Intensification of cow/calf production: a history. In: Range beef cow Symposium. 2001. p. 91.

2. Taylor RE. Historical landmarks in the American Cattle Industry. In: Beef production and management decisions. New York: Macmillan; 1994. p. 559–68.

3. Arthur PF. Double muscling in cattle: a review. Aust J Agric Res 1995;46: 1493–515.

4. Gregory KE, Echternkamp SE, Cundiff LV. Effects of twinning on dystocia, calf survival, calf growth, carcass traits, and cow productivity. J Anim Sci 1996; 74(6):1223–33.
5. Rice LE. Dystocia-related risk factors. Vet Clin North Am 1994;10(1):53–68.
6. Saad HM, Thomas MG, Speidel SE, et al. Differential response from selection for high calving ease vs. low birth weight in American Simmental beef cattle. J Anim Sci 2020;98(7):162.
7. Rogers RW, Martin SW, Meek AH. Reproductive efficiency and calf survival in Ontario beef cow-calf herds: a cross-sectional mail survey. Can J Comp Med 1985; 49:27–33.
8. Martin SW, Schwabe CW, Franti CE. Dairy calf mortality rate: influence of management and housing factors on calf mortality in Tulare County, California. Am J Vet Res 1975;36(08):1111–4.
9. Townsend HGG. Environmental factors and calving management practices that affect neonatal mortality in the beef calf. Vet Clin North Am 1994;10(1):119–26.
10. Schumann FJ, Townsend HG, Naylor JM, et al. Risk factors for mortality from diarrhea in beef calves in Alberta. Can J Vet Res 1990;54:366–72.
11. Clement JC, King ME, Wittum TE, et al. Factors associated with the incidence of calf scours in North Dakota Beef herds. Agri-Practice 1993;14:13–7.
12. Clement JC, King ME, Wittum TE, et al. Use of epidemiologic principles to identify risk factors associated with the development of diarrhea in calves in five beef herds. J Am Vet Med Assoc 1995;287:1334–8.
13. Pence M, Robbe S, Thomson JU. Reducing the incidence of neonatal calf diarrhea through evidence-based management. Compend 2001;S73–5.
14. Snodgrass DR. Evaluation of a combined rotavirus and enterotoxigenic Escherichia coli vaccine in cattle. Vet Rec 1986;119:39–42.
15. Cornaglia EM, Fernandez FM, Gottschalk M, et al. Reduction in morbidity due to diarrhea in nursing beef calves by use of an inactivated oil-adjuvanted rotavirus – Escherischia coli vaccine in the dam. Vet Microbiol 1992;30:191–202.
16. Bendali F, Sanaa M, Bichet H, et al. Risk factors associated with diarrhea in newborn calves. Vet Res 1999;30:509–22.
17. Garry F. Differentiating causes of neonatal calf enteritis to enhance management and prevention. Bov Pract 2020;53:165–9.
18. Atwill ER, Johnson EM, Pereira MG. Association of herd composition, stocking rate, and duration of calving season with fecal shedding of Cryptosporidium parvum oocysts in beef herds. J Am Vet Med Assoc 1999;215:1833–8.
19. Smith DR, Grotelueschen DM, Knott T, et al. Population dynamics of undifferentiated neonatal calf diarrhea among ranch beef calves. Bov Pract 2008;42:1.
20. Smith DR, Grotelueschen DM, Knott T, et al. Strategies for controlling neonatal diarrhea in cow-calf herds–the Sandhills calving system. AABP Proc 2006; 39:94–8.
21. Smith DR, Grotelueschen D, Knott T, et al. Managing to alleviate calf scours: the Sandhills calving system. In: Range beef cow Symposium. 2003. p. 70.
22. King Ranch Institute for Ranch Management, TX A&M Univ. John B. Armstrong Lectureship on Systems Thinking, Aug. 12-15, 2019.

Wellness Management in Beef Feeder Cattle

Changing Mental Models to Support Beneficial Emergent System Behaviors

T. Robin Falkner, DVM[a,b,]*

KEYWORDS

- Systems thinking • Bovine respiratory disease (BRD) • Wellness • Well-being
- Mental model • Sickness behavior • Treatment success • imal welfare

KEY POINTS

- Mental models, or paradigms, guide and constrain perspective as cognitive biases, are often unrecognized, and are difficult to change.
- Current animal health mental models are grounded in sickness (or failure) perspectives instead of wellness (or success) perspectives.
- Improvements in animal health diagnosis and clinical outcomes can be achieved by managing wellness outcomes as continuous variables instead of for the dichotomous absence of failure outcomes.
- Improved management of wellness outcomes creates a common ground and shared vision between production medicine objectives and animal welfare expectations.
- The concept of managing for improvements in success outcomes instead of the absence of failure outcomes can be broadly expanded by veterinarians into a new Systems Practice paradigm.

INTRODUCTION: SICKNESS-BIASED PARADIGMS/MENTAL MODELS

One of the foundational underpinnings of Donella Meadows' *Thinking in Systems: A Primer*[1] is that mental models[2] exert the highest leverage points in a system. This is also represented in Iceberg Models, where the base of the iceberg is Mental Models, described as the values, assumptions, and beliefs that guide or constrain perspective.[3] In *Leverage Points*,[4] Meadows emphasized the high leverage of changing the goals of a system and transcending existing, constraining paradigms. Kuhn, in the seminal 1962 book *The Structure of Scientific Revolutions*,[5] first

[a] CattleFlow Consulting, Christiana, TN 37037, USA; [b] Elanco Animal Health, Greenfield, IN, USA
* 2404 Walnut Grove Road, Christiana, TN 37037.
E-mail address: rfalkner@bellsouth.net

Vet Clin Food Anim 38 (2022) 273–294
https://doi.org/10.1016/j.cvfa.2022.02.007
0749-0720/22/© 2022 Elsevier Inc. All rights reserved.

proposed that significant advancements in science usually resulted from what he termed paradigm shifts instead of steady progress within the current paradigm, and that when progress slows and anomalies to current paradigms accrue, a paradigm shift should follow. There are ongoing discussions in human medicine around current paradigms representing "sick care" rather than "health care" mental models, calling for changes from reductionist approaches on sickness to systems approaches on health, and for medical curricula to "emphasize homeostasis and health rather than only disease and diagnosis."[6] These discussions were stimulated by the anomaly of declining human health outcomes despite rising costs and investments in the sickness paradigm.

New mental models can help one see new things previously present but unrecognized, interpret old information in new ways, and provide new insights from new perspectives, but existing mental models tend to be deeply ingrained and inflexible frameworks that are difficult to recognize and change.[7] Mental models function as comfortable, silent cognitive biases that limit perspective. However, systems science, and in particular systems modeling, provides insight into existing mental models and means to explore potential improvements in perspective.

It is proposed that animal health, and in particular beef cattle veterinary practice, shares a sickness-focused paradigm with human medicine: Unacceptable outcomes exhibiting refractoriness to the current sickness paradigm, such as steadily increasing losses to bovine respiratory disease (BRD),[8,9] are anomalies that point to the potential for new wellness paradigms to emerge.

This article provides an example of the utility of systems methodology to beef veterinarians wishing to combine research insights, client system knowledge, and experience into management hypotheses to first refine and test with systems models before evaluating in production systems. A primary purpose of modeling system behaviors is to make better informed decisions in complex systems, often where research studies do not provide much guidance. The example involves a change in mental model from sickness to wellness perspective.

TERMINOLOGY

Words that are interpreted differently by author and reader are problematic. Health is defined by *Merriam-Webster* as "the condition of being well or free of disease."[10] The first statement in the preamble of the constitution of the World Health Organization (WHO),[11] unchanged since 1948, is more expansive: "Health is a state of complete physical, mental and social well-being and not merely the absence of disease or infirmity." In 2001, a US presidential council[12] addressed the definition of wellness: "wellness is multidimensional; wellness is a state of being described as positive health; wellness is part of health; wellness is possessed by the individual; quality of life and wellbeing are the descriptors of wellness; and health and its positive component (wellness) are integrated." There is considerable inconsistency in the common usage of all associated terminology. The common use of the phrase "animal health and welfare," including in the veterinarian's oath,[13] suggests the term "animal health" is often used and understood in the Merriam-Webster definition as "free of disease." Wellness and well-being can be similarly confusing in usage and interpretation. For the purposes of this article, wellness will be used consistent with the WHO definition of health and the presidential council's definition of wellness, as a "positive component of health." This will allow the reader to retain any preexisting concept of health and interpret the use of wellness herein as a positive spectrum of health existing on a continuum beyond the mere absence of sickness of infirmity.

DEVELOPING A WELLNESS MENTAL MODEL

Wellness is used in this article not as sickness antonym but as a construct of well-being independent of disease status. Well-being is associated with positive observable wellness behaviors,[14] and researchers have found reduced wellness behavior expression has utility as an early indication of diseases like mastitis[15] and metritis.[16] However, there is also ample evidence that common management systems such as confinement[17] and practices such as castration[18] can reduce expression of wellness behaviors in the absence of disease. In this article, a systems approach is used to explore potential animal health implications of management systems and practices that improve both animal expression and human observation of wellness, specifically, improving the early and accurate identification and judicious treatment of disease. In addition, a process for transitioning mental model from a linear, reductive focus on managing disease outcomes to a more holistic systems perspective managing emergent systems properties supporting wellness outcomes is illustrated. Fortuitously, increased focus on wellness could simultaneously improve production outcomes while providing better alignment with emerging animal welfare paradigms.[19]

CURRENT MENTAL MODELS

Veterinarians often struggle to define and manage animal health along a continuum of success outcomes versus as simply the absence of failure outcomes. The daily routine is filled with treating negative outcomes or trying to prevent them: morbidity, mortality, open cows, performance loss, and negative welfare states. This perspective likely supports a flawed dichotomy where the absence of failure is interpreted as success. Veterinarians usually measure and manage failure breakpoints even when communicating them in success terms. For example, if one communicates in terms of BRD success, it does not fundamentally change an underlying dichotomous mental model focused on morbidity, treatment failure, and mortality outcomes.

Transitioning to a wellness perspective creates quite a challenge, for one will find few existing constructs by which animal health outcomes are measured, discussed, and managed as continuous wellness variables instead of at dichotomous failure breakpoints. **Fig. 1** demonstrates a dichotomous sickness mental model where success is the absence of failure.

Managing BRD is limited by the low sensitivity of clinical diagnosis. Researchers found lung lesions in twice as many cattle as were treated for BRD, indicating many animals with BRD were never identified and treated.[20] The prevalence of lung lesions in cattle never identified as sick approached that of cattle with a history of treatment. Others found similar lung lesions at harvest in treated and untreated animals.[21,22] A meta-analysis of 7 studies found the sensitivity of BRD diagnosis was low (0.27; 95% Confidence Interval: CI: 0.12–0.65).[23] From a judicious use perspective, the absence of disease evidence in many treated animals is also problematic. The apparent low accuracy of disease detection presents the critical systems question, "how can BRD diagnosis be improved?"

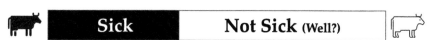

Logical Fallacy:
If sickness is the expression of disease, then wellness is absence of sickness

Fig. 1. Dichotomous pass/fail mental model.

There are several potential explanations for difficulty in accurately diagnosing BRD, which include the propensity of prey species to mask the symptoms of illness.[24] In addition, there is a large overlap between sickness behaviors and stress behaviors, and a negative impact of stress on wellness behavior expression.[25] BRD most often occurs in the immediate postweaning or postarrival period[26] when animals transition into a new production segment, and this transition is accompanied by stressors like weaning, transport, handling, painful management procedures, vaccination, new environment, adaptation to new feedstuffs, social stress from confinement, and disruption of social structure.

Stress programming[27] or chronic stress[28] resulting from sequential and novel stressors can negatively impact immunologic function[29] and program negative judgment bias.[30] Negativity bias, observed as a negative judgment bias or pessimism toward novel experiences, has been studied in relation to animal welfare.[31] Pessimism can follow negative experiences associated with fear, stress, or pain, although individual animal differences also exist.[32] In chronically stressed sheep, adding positive experiences to a chronic stress model was shown to induce a positive bias or optimism state.[33] Of particular interest in disease diagnosis was an increase in the frequency in which the lambs approached a human, which could make them easier to observe and less likely to mask sickness behaviors from caretakers.

Modeling (**Fig. 2**) suggests an innate or induced negativity bias could power a vicious cycle wherein benign and/or novel experiences are interpreted as threatening, resulting in the creation of system reinforcing loops for both additional negativity bias and stress. The modeled potential of providing more positive experiences to mitigate, or balance, negative ones present in production settings deserves further study.

An important lesson from the modeled structure of the stress/negativity bias causal loop diagram (CLD) in **Fig. 2** is that it is self-reinforcing and may be balanced by positive experiences. This supports a mental model of wellness existing along a positive continuum instead of only in the reduction of negatives. A stressed animal is

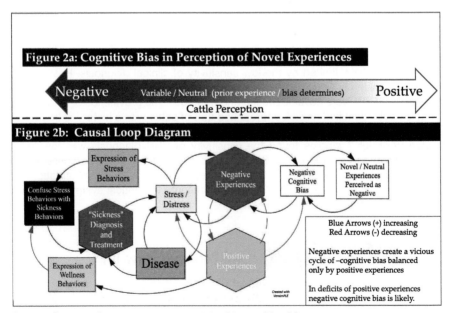

Fig. 2. Influence of experiences on cognitive bias and health outcomes.

predisposed to exhibit stress behaviors easily confused with sickness behaviors, mask sickness behaviors from its caretakers, and show diminished wellness behaviors in the absence of disease. Research in cattle and swine has demonstrated the attitudes and behaviors of a stockperson impact animal behaviors, performance, and reproductive success.[34–36]

INSIGHT FROM RECENT STUDIES ON SICKNESS BEHAVIORS IN FEEDER CATTLE

A recent dissertation[37] on BRD sickness behavior provides insight into the potential impact of stress from management and management systems on the expression of wellness behaviors and incidence of BRD in feeder cattle. In 3 included studies, beef calves from a university herd were used. The designs were likely stressful, requiring daily animal removal and handling in a chute for clinical scoring over 12- to 15-day periods. In study 1, weaned beef calves were acclimated to the research feedlot for 9 weeks before administering a BRD challenge model. In the study, 5/10 unchallenged controls developed spontaneous BRD over the 14-day observation and had to be excluded from analysis. In study 2, there was no acclimation between arrival at the facility and BRD challenge, and 5/20 unchallenged controls developed spontaneous BRD over a 15-day observation. In study 3, naturally occurring BRD in the period immediately postarrival was used instead of the challenge model. A spontaneous BRD morbidity of 31% (25/80) occurred over a 12-day observation period in calves that under commercial conditions would probably be considered (the author's opinion) at relatively low risk for BRD: single-source, prevaccinated for BRD pathogens as part of complete health program, preweaned for greater than 30 days at farm of origin, acclimated to bunks and feed, and transported only 84 km directly to facility.

A relevant challenge to current dogma is posed by the high spontaneous BRD in the short study observation periods: "is BRD risk primarily a quality possessed by a calf accountable to the cow/calf producer, or an emergent property of the system it enters upon leaving its birth herd and accountable to that system?" In study 1, in calves that were acclimated in the facility for 9 weeks, execution of the study protocol resulted in 50% morbidity in 2 weeks in unchallenged controls. In study 3, "preconditioned" calves experienced 31% spontaneous BRD within 14 days of arrival.

The utility of BRD sickness metrics across the studies was consistent, but grooming activity, a wellness behavior, was not. In study 1, with acclimated cattle, grooming behavior was present and had predictive utility for BRD diagnosis. In study 2 and 3, with unacclimated cattle, it did not. The researcher adds that study 3 might more closely resemble commercial conditions and was disappointed grooming activity did not have utility in BRD diagnosis. Comparison of the provided graphs provides insight. In study 1, grooming activity was present and declined in nonmorbid unchallenged calves subjected to study handling stress but by more in challenged animals. In study 3, nonmorbid animals had low to no grooming activity to lose when stricken with spontaneous BRD. The author of this article proposes that the management system, including study execution, did not support wellness sufficiently for nonmorbid calves to exhibit grooming behavior in study 3 and that the stress imposed by the feedlot/study system was likely the key factor in spontaneous BRD morbidity. Other management systems providing a less stressful transition could provide different results on grooming behavior and improved BRD outcomes. A relevant, unstudied research question posed would be "are low observed wellness behaviors in the immediate post arrival period indicative of stress-inducing cattle and management system mismatches and/or predictive of BRD risk?"

MANAGING ADMIXTURES OF ANIMAL BEHAVIORAL EXPRESSION

During the period of highest BRD incidence, an admixture of stressed and sick animals could result in missed or late treatments in sick animals and stressed animals being misdiagnosed as sick and treated (**Fig. 3**). Misdiagnosis of illness leads to inaccurate health management records, reduced true treatment success rates (often concealed by excessive treatment of nonmorbid animals), additional stress from unnecessary treatments, wastage of labor resources needed to provide virtuous husbandry, and nonjudicious antimicrobial use.

Fig. 3 identifies a critical system leverage point for improving the accuracy of BRD diagnosis is managing for wellness behaviors so nonmorbid animals are not express-ing stress behaviors that can confound accurate and timely diagnosis. In addition to the benefits already mentioned, decreased stress decreases susceptibility to BRD,[38] and Hazard stated that "stress should be thought of as a disease because it is probably the precursor to many of the viral and bacterial infections that make up the bovine respiratory disease syndrome". Additionally, any caretaker resources spared by elimination of unnecessary treatment of nonmorbid animals could be applied to beneficial activities that increase husbandry and positive animal experi-ences. Longer term, the efficacy of therapeutics might be preserved through less and more judicious use.[39,40]An additional perspective is that a stressed animal mis-diagnosed and treated for BRD early in the management period might receive a less efficacious treatment if diagnosed with BRD later. An illustrative example of the underrecognized utility of better managing wellness expression is provided in **Box 1**.

TOOLS TO PROACTIVELY MANAGE WELLNESS

An extensive review was conducted of clinical illness scoring (CIS) heuristics and emerging technologies, such as remote temperature sensing, thermography, behavior monitoring, and computer-aided auscultation used in BRD management that is not included here. The reader is referred to another review[41] and examples.[42,43] The re-view revealed a common denominator in application of a sickness paradigm perspec-tive to obtain a dichotomous answer to the question "Treat for BRD?," whether a simple "temp and treat" at feedlot arrival or highly sophisticated behavior monitoring

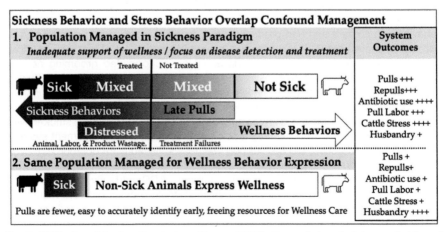

Fig. 3. Difficulty of Bovine Respiratory Disease (BRD) diagnosis in admixtures of sick and stressed animals.

Box 1
Wellness insight from a master cattleman

My mentor and feeder cattle management author, Dr Gordon Hazard, provided me early insight on wellness behaviors. As I was learning BRD diagnosis under his tutelage, he questioned my picking a calf that coughed, "Do you not see the nine lick marks (self-grooming) on its side?" When I identified a calf separated from the herd as a BRD suspect, he immediately concluded the calf was not sick. When asked how he knew with a quick glance from such distance, he replied he had seen the calf rise and stretch earlier. Years later, those calves came back to mind, but in new perspective. If subsets of calves were exhibiting clear sickness or wellness behaviors that day, what were the rest of the animals? Difficult to diagnose accurately! In many feeder cattle systems, a majority of calves might exhibit a confusing behavioral stressed-but-not-sick diagnostic dilemma at some point after arrival, confounding accurage and timely diagnosis. The wellness paradigm breakthrough came from a new question: "Can we manage to get more nonmorbid cattle to exhibit stronger wellness behaviors?" I, like most, was focused on preventing, diagnosing and treating disease (failure) and missed the management utility in understanding and managing for better expression of wellness behaviors (success). Often in systems that poorly supported this outcome. Not only was wellness's potential unrealized but any negative implications of my management recommendations on wellness behaviors were inadequately considered.

---

systems. No examples were found of proactive management of wellness behaviors on a continuum above a disease or infirmity set breakpoint. The design and conduct of studies to explore the utility of managing wellness in system success perspective instead of individual animal failure await the emergence of a wellness paradigm and systems science in animal health research. This does not preclude a practitioner, with accountability for outcomes, from exploring wellness management in client systems.

WELFARE IMPLICATIONS

Positive wellness behaviors include activities like self-grooming, positive social interactions, inquisitiveness, play, and positive cognitive bias in response to novel or benign experiences.[44] Although there is considerable individual variation in these behaviors, a given animal will likely exhibit more wellness behaviors as comfort level and sense of security increase. Although managing to support wellness behaviors is presented here primarily for its management utility instead of an association with animal welfare, there is evolving perspective in animal welfare along a parallel axis. Various proposals to update the "5 Freedoms of Animal Welfare" (5F)[45] developed in the 1960s have been adopted. The 5F's were "freedom from … (negative experiences and states)." The emergent view is animal welfare should include promotion of positive experiences and states, not just freedom from negative ones. The 5 Provisions (5P)[46] and 5 Domains (5D)[19] are examples of movement to welfare guidelines that include provision for animals positively exhibiting wellness. Domain 4 of the 5D, named Behavioral Interactions, includes animals consciously seeking specific goals and exhibiting wellness behaviors when interacting with (1) environment, (2) other animals and (3) humans. Domain 5 is assessment of mental state. The recent adoption of the 5D by a large beef processor[47] could presage increasing expectations of positive wellness outcomes in supply chains. When considered along with benefits of positive psychological states on physical health,[48] the physiologic mechanisms of which are extensively studied,[49] and utility in improving cattle management proposed in this article, veterinarians should need little encouragement to begin the transition of mental and management models into positive wellness perspectives.

MODELING WELLNESS IN A COMPLEX ADAPTIVE SYSTEM

In the following section, examples are presented and may represent either mental or systems models. A model for managing any outcome includes awareness of the components influencing the outcome. A crucial understanding is that complex systems are not modeled with traditional parts from the disassembly of wholes by reductive science in a facsimile of a blueprint. In systems thinking, power is in modeling behavior, particularly emergent systems behavior (ESB) that is not a quality of any part. Most biological systems are complex adaptive systems and generate ESBs.[50] Although often discussed from the perspective of unexpected and/or unwanted outcomes, ESBs are also the path to creating system properties that do not exist as properties of individual parts. In prominent examples from this article, the objective is to model an ESB of "support of accurate and timely BRD diagnosis," which contains other ESBs, including "expression and communication of wellness." Such a model can be visualized using a CLD.[1] Additional ESB examples are feed intake, stress, wellness expression, employee engagement, and biocontainment.

ESBs cannot be purchased as products and added to a system to produce results; they are holistic system properties resulting from structure, feedback, and the complex interaction of parts.[50] In reductive and product-centric mental and systems models, one tends to overemphasize tangible parts and create parts lists or blueprints.

PART 1: LINEAR MENTAL/SYSTEMS MODELS

For example, a common mental model of vaccination and wellness often consists of a simple linear model (LM; **Fig. 4**).

This LM has no no utility in understanding how vaccination interacts with other parts within a system. It fails as a causal model because vaccination does not cause health. In linear modeling, arrows are often drawn between components that simply have some relationship. In causal models, the arrows have a second quality: they either increase or decrease the following component. In application of the linear mental model, there is an implied arrow (dashed red) going from Health back to Vaccination: Poor Health → Vaccine changes. In application, this flawed LM may be inappropriately used as a CLD. In such use, poor health feeds back for more vaccination or vaccine changes because vaccines are seen as containing the property of health. This mental model not only biases for the diagnosis of vaccine deficiencies but also usually presumes disease as principally pathogen-caused instead of with more complex underlying cause. An important additional perspective is that one can add a large amount of

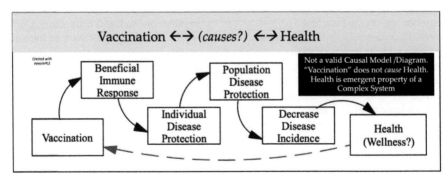

Fig. 4. Vaccinology linear mental/systems model.

reductive detail and knowledge in immunology, vaccines, and epidemiology to this mental model without changing the shortcomings of the construct: vaccination → causes → health. The potential value of additional knowledge is compromised by the flawed paradigm that constrains it.

PART 2: LINEAR-BASED SYSTEM-OF-SYSTEM MODELS

Typically, reductive mental models take multiple LMs and assemble broader systems perspectives from them. **Fig. 5** represents the assembly of LM subassemblies into a feeder calf system or mental model for Health. This model is maybe best considered a linear system of systems[51] because subassemblies are viewed primarily as working independently of each other and adding together into Health sums. Given that the underlying LM subassemblies like "Vaccinology" have issues, it might be anticipated that a linear combination of these subcomponents is also flawed.

The diagram typifies a flawed "Health is the sum of the system parts" mental model in a pile of parts with lack of structure. It also demonstrates causation failure. There is no nutritional value in Parasite Control, therefore it cannot cause Nutrition (gray arrow). Whenever the LM arrows are not strongly causative, it may conceal a component or valuable ESB awaiting discovery.

PART 3: CAUSAL MODELING AND IDENTIFICATION OF EMERGENT SYSTEMS BEHAVIOR

Transitioning into causal modeling is demonstrated in **Fig. 6**. Parasitism is modeled to cause reduction in Feed Intake, which causes reduced Nutritional Status. Feed Intake becomes the first ESB in the model other than Health. It was located by making the structure in **Fig. 5** causal instead of simply relational. Discovery of this ESB led to recognizing an additional leverageable ESB it supports, Wellness Behaviors, and it to another, Accuracy BRD Diagnosis. However, it is unlikely the potential of this ESB of ESBs would be linearly modeled into: it would need to be identified first, and if valuable, modeled for. Such insight can dramatically change the selection of and assembly of parts because the contribution of individual parts to ESBs might be more

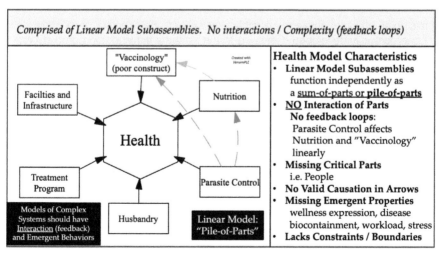

Fig. 5. Illustrative linear system-of-system mental model.

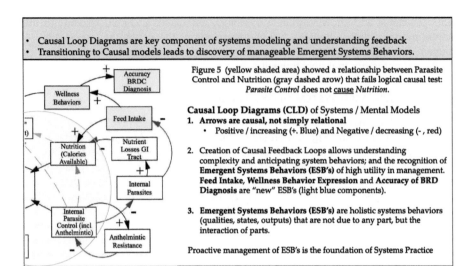

* Causal Loop Diagrams are key component of systems modeling and understanding feedback
* Transitioning to Causal models leads to discovery of manageable Emergent Systems Behaviors.

Figure 5 (yellow shaded area) showed a relationship between Parasite Control and Nutrition (gray dashed arow) that fails logical causal test: *Parasite Control* does not <u>cause</u> *Nutrition*.

Causal Loop Diagrams (CLD) of Systems / Mental Models
1. **Arrows are causal, not simply relational**
   * Positive / increasing (+. Blue) and Negative / decreasing (- , red)

2. Creation of Causal Feedback Loops allows understanding complexity and anticipating system behaviors; and the recognition of **Emergent Systems Behaviors (ESB's)** of high utility in management. **Feed Intake, Wellness Behavior Expression** and **Accuracy of BRD Diagnosis** are "new" ESB's (light blue components).

3. **Emergent Systems Behaviors (ESB's)** are holistic systems behaviors (qualities, states, outputs) that are not due to any part, but the interaction of parts.

Proactive management of ESB's is the foundation of Systems Practice

Fig. 6. Transitioning linear, relational mental models to causal models.

important than their previously recognized primary properties. As an example, the vaccine X might be more efficacious in a challenge model than vaccine Z, but also cause more stress and injection site reactions and be less trusted by purchasers of feeder cattle. The additional immunologic properties of vaccine X may have far less total system value than the ancillary properties of vaccine Z. Finally, care must be taken in not forcing ESBs back into a linear paradigm: A product that made every animal, including sick animals, exhibit wellness would have negative implications on BRD management. One might not only be reducing symptoms of disease that have disease benefits, like fever,[25] but also interfering with the important ESB of accurate and timely BRD diagnosis.

WELLNESS CAUSAL LOOP MODELING CAUSAL LOOP MODELING OF WELLNESS VERSUS SICKNESS

At this point, an interesting and plausible new wellness perspective, or mental model, has been partially developed. Referring to the systems thinking and paradigm references,[1–5,7] changes in mental model (or paradigm) exert the highest leverage in a system. The foundation of the new paradigm is that wellness is not simply the dichotomous absence of sickness, but a broader continuum that exists when disease is not present. A potential high utility of increased expression of wellness behaviors in nonmorbid animals in improving BRD diagnosis has also been supported (see **Fig. 3**). In **Fig. 7**, wellness outcomes are modeled as separate from sickness outcomes, interacting through constructs of Stress and Wellness Resources/Support. The wellness component creates a different structure than models created in disease perspective, where wellness is unmodeled as the absence of sickness.[52]

At this point, ignore the animal health product inputs to the left in **Fig. 7**. Exploring the structure and interactions within the main model reveals interesting behavior: Disease functions in a reinforcing, vicious cycle with Stress, while Wellness works in a balancing, virtuous manner to decrease Stress and Disease. In addition, Disease reinforces itself through the Wellness Resources /Support loop. The net result is that Disease Outcomes function in vicious cycles to increase Disease Outcomes by both

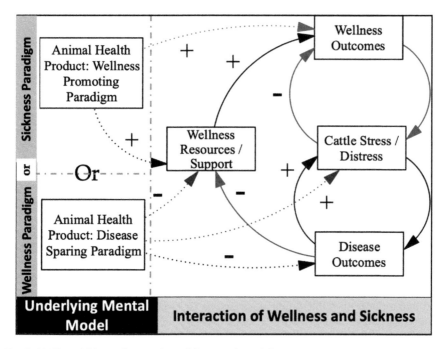

Fig. 7. Wellness/sickness interaction with mental model.

increasing Stress in the system and consuming Wellness Resources. The only balancing of sickness is wellness. Simply stated, the process of treating disease or misdiagnosed stress behaviors is stressful to the animal and peers and consumes resources that could be used to support wellness.

Accepting the basic wellness premises of the **Fig. 7** model but remaining in the sickness mental model demonstrated in **Fig. 4** is problematic. In **Fig. 4**, an animal health product was viewed as causing wellness. When this underlying sickness-product paradigm/mental model is retained, the function of **Fig. 7** is demonstrated in the upper left quadrant. When faced with a need to improve wellness, the mental model signals for additional application of products seen as containing the property wellness. This is contrasted with the wellness mental model demonstrated in the lower left quadrant. In this wellness mental model, the vaccine is not seen as containing the property wellness, but as having potential disease-sparing properties positive for wellness, but also as potentially increasing Stress and decreasing Wellness Resources. An example of mental model failure occurs when a sickness practitioner finds the presence of an organism and adds a booster or revaccination to the protocol. This might result in improved immunity but would also result in any wellness compromising effects like stress from the product or additional cattle handling. Also, the human resources required for the booster could be diverted from other activities, potentially including those that directly support wellness, like husbandry. In addition, the negativity cognitive bias or Pessimism CLD in **Fig. 2** comes into play with an added booster vaccination. Two negative events, an additional cattle handling and vaccine response, are added, possibly at the cost of positive experiences, such as simply being around the cattle in a nonthreatening posture or performing husbandry activities. Insight from the negativity cognitive bias model (see **Fig. 2**) suggests utility in increasing positive interactions and decreasing negative ones, and this is likely a metric to consider managing both in direct accounting of interactions and in measured wellness outcomes.

LITERATURE SUPPORT OF UTILITY OF MODELING ANIMAL HEALTH PRODUCTS AS DISEASE-SPARING INSTEAD OF WELLNESS-PROMOTING

There is a considerable body of literature supporting that vaccinations should not be viewed as possessing wellness properties, but instead as having both disease sparing and wellness-compromising properties. Both a meta-analysis[53] and broad review[54] found limited utility or efficiency of vaccination for BRD in arriving feeder calves. There are also studies demonstrating negative effects of vaccines. Stokka and colleagues[55] found clostridial vaccination increased acute phase proteins and decreased feed intake. Baccili and colleagues,[56] using dairy heifers, demonstrated significant systemic inflammatory responses from viral vaccines. Of particular interest is that the adjuvanted vaccines eliciting greater humoral antibody responses produced greater systemic inflammatory responses, worsening with subsequent doses, suggesting higher efficacy may come at a cost of higher undesirable effects. Tizard states[57] that Bovine Viral Diarrhea Virus (BVDV) vaccines can suppress neutrophil function and lymphocyte blastogenesis and potentially exacerbate concurrent infections: and that modified-live (MLV) Infectious Bovine Rhinotracheitis Virus (IBRV) vaccines exacerbate experimental *Moraxella bovis* pinkeye. Griebel[58] noted field reports of postvaccinal MLVBVDV immunosuppression, and Richeson et al e[59] found reduced white blood cell counts in feeder calves administered MLVBVDV vaccine on arrival. A BVDV review by Waltz and colleagues[60] for the American College of Veterinary Internal Medicine produced the following consensus statement: "Evidence that BVDV vaccination decreases naturally occurring BRD complex in field settings is limited and of low quality." A well-replicated field study found delaying viral vaccination until after the highest BRD risk period reduced the number of animals requiring 2 or more BRD treatments.[61] A recent study with negative and positive injectable vaccine controls demonstrated intranasal vaccine-associated increases in the nasal carriage of *Histophilus somni*, a BRD pathogen.[62] A meta-analysis of studies containing negative controls found delaying BRD vaccines in arriving feeder cattle did not change health outcomes[63] even though delaying vaccination would seem to decrease potential vaccine efficiency because BRD risk is greatest in the immediate postarrival period. The cited references should not be taken to reflect an antivaccine bias of the author or cited researchers. To the contrary, the author believes vaccines are one of the most important tools in the animal health arsenal, used correctly, and recommends them in feeder cattle systems (it is hoped, correctly, but without a fixed protocol because individual systems can vary greatly in what correctly might be). The author is confident also that use can produce negative wellness consequences in complex systems, and that any mental model that prioritizes more and more potent vaccination in feeder cattle systems as a certain path to more wellness will find little evidence-based support.

The mental models misconstruing vaccines as possessing wellness qualities can extend to other animal health products. Few product uses have demonstrated more consistent efficiency in field trials than antimicrobials used for BRD control.[64] However, an antimicrobial likely does not contain wellness properties, but disease-sparing ones. The literature supports that antimicrobial use can also be accompanied by undesirable outcomes. Although studies of antimicrobial effects on the feeder cattle biome are uncommon, a study in young calves demonstrated genus-level differences and less bacterial diversity in those exposed to antimicrobials.[65] In dairy cattle, the systemic use of certain antimicrobials, and not others, was associated with increased prevalence of antimicrobial-resistant non-aureus *Staphylococci* in the udder microbiota.[66] Snyder and colleagues[67] reported an increase in the carriage of multidrug-resistant (MDR) BRD bacteria in high-risk feeder calves from 3.7% on arrival, when tulathromycin was administered, to 99.2% 14 days later, and called for more research on the impact of antimicrobial use on MDR and MDR on morbidity and mortality. In a subsequent review on antimicrobial resistance in cattle, Credille[68] summarized research on *Mannheimia haemolytica* in cattle as suggesting some uses might be driving resistance, primarily by enabling the propagation of strains with acquired MDR integrative conjugative elements (ICE), seen as especially problematic because ICE can be transferred between BRD-associated bacteria. In a study conducted in healthy feedlot cattle, administration of an antimicrobial caused a reduction in feed intake compared with negative controls.[69] Antimicrobials are likely among the most impactful animal health products used in many feeder cattle systems, following only management and husbandry in disease outcome mitigation, but there is still much to learn about how to apply them best and sustainably across diverse production systems.

A more exhaustive review is not necessary to conclude that the use of any animal health product in a complex system can create unexpected and/or unwanted effects. Some of them, like antimicrobial resistance, might be delayed in emerging and have significant future consequences. The potential for long-term positive ESBs is as unrecognized as negative ESBs are unanticipated. Current production research models, which primarily measure short-term performance outcomes, are not designed nor conducted to measure future emergent outcomes or immediate emergent behaviors, such as ease and accuracy of BRD diagnosis. External validity of studies or experience across complex systems that may consist of similar parts but different structures, interactions, and emergent behaviors is difficult to assess. Clinical observation is possibly the most powerful tool in ascertaining emergent or delayed behaviors in individual complex systems. Sound systems modeling can better anticipate and assist in understanding such behaviors.

The literature supports the perspective that in complex biological systems with emergent behaviors an animal health product with clear benefits in the prevention, control, or treatment of disease can influence other outcomes, some immediate and some emergent and delayed, that may or may not be desirable. Better understanding complex interactions and behavior in production systems would allow products to be used with more efficiency and sustainability. Viewing products with efficiency in disease reduction through a mental model that biases them to health promoting instead of disease sparing is seriously limited in perspective. One question arising is "what about a product that reduces the use of wellness supporting resources such as a treatment that requires fewer doses and less animal handling, is that not wellness promoting?" The answer is no, the product is still not wellness promoting, just potentially less wellness compromising than an alternative requiring more treatments.

A MORE COMPLETE SYSTEMS WELLNESS MODEL

The first sections of this article functioned to build and support a reasonable hypothesis that managing to improve expression of wellness behaviors in nonmorbid cattle has utility in improving BRD outcomes. Lacking research studies examining this question directly, models were constructed to better understand the interaction of systems parts to produce wellness outcomes on a continuum. To allow more direct comparisons to other systems models of BRD that exclude wellness except as the absence of sickness, **Fig. 8** is also provided. It is not complete, but allows more insight into the complex interactions occurring outside of those modeled in **Fig. 7**, including those components the author feels are most important to understanding behavior in feeder cattle systems:

1. Business model awareness
2. People outcomes
3. Animal wellness support
4. Biocontainment
5. Disease outcomes
6. Performance outcomes
7. System properties like resilience, robustness, and sustainability

Some of the system subassemblies, like business model and biocontainment, are complex and need their own models not included here. It would be impossible to fully explain **Fig. 8** within the limitations of this format. The model contains a large amount of information that may be of value to those who conclude at this point that transitioning to a wellness paradigm has value. Additional study, investing in acquiring knowledge on systems thinking and systems modeling, particularly CLDs and emergence, is suggested.

There is tremendous value in modeling as a learning activity, and it exemplifies an iterative process in use and supports a continuous improvement mindset. The systems thinking perspective is more one of outcomes management than problem solving

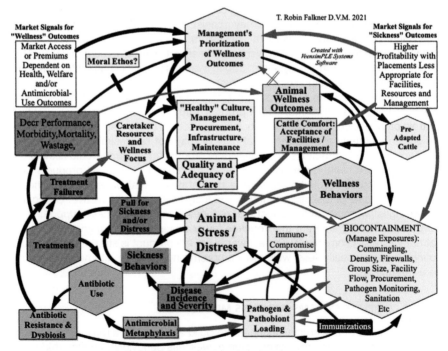

"Hexagons" have highest "First Principle" leverage on "Wellness Outcomes". Key: Blue Arrows (+) "increasing". Red Arrows (-) "decreasing". COMPARTMENTS: Light Blue: System Wellness Inputs. Light Green:-System Wellness Outcomes. Yellow: System Disease/Distress Inputs. Pink: System Sickness Outcomes. Gray: Antimicrobial Use. White: Market Signals.

Fig. 8. Wellness outcomes in US feeder cattle system(s).

because the systems will exhibit emergent behavior, and yesterday's solution often becomes part of tomorrow's problem even when sound systems thinking principles and modeling are used. Do not expect off-the-shelf models to provide ongoing utility needed across diverse client systems with steady emergence of new behaviors that frustrate the old model. With improved systems perspective, management systems once considered similar based on parts content become dissimilar when different structures, constraints, boundaries, and unique emergent qualities are recognized.

Key components with high leverage are represented in the model as hexagons, (1) exhibition of wellness behavior, (2) biocontainment, (3) caretaker resources, (4) management priorities (5) stress, (6) number of treatments performed, and (7) antimicrobial use.

Similarly, components were grouped by color coding into key compartments to allow better visualization. Importantly, disease outcomes (pink) were separated from wellness outcomes (green) to reflect rejection of the dichotomous perspective of wellness as absence of disease. Other components interact through functional compartments represented as wellness inputs (blue), disease inputs (yellow), antimicrobial use (gray), and market signals (white). Notable is the inclusion of new parts like people and deemphasizing prominent LM parts. There is also intent in getting the causal arrows to represent true communication and flow of information when possible. The deemphasis of animal health products as pro-wellness and modeling instead as disease-mitigating with influence on other emergent behaviors is consistent with the new wellness mental model.

Fig. 8 omits important parts of the management system such as nutrition that interact with the included components but are not necessary here. This is not the same as inferring nutrition does not matter in wellness, it simply is not needed here to visualize emergent behaviors like stress, wellness, disease, antimicrobial resistance, and the BRD diagnostic accuracy of particular interest.

By following the flows through the system, understanding interconnections and feedback loops, it becomes evident that this system has some unique qualities, particularly as concerns emergent behavior. Increasing focus on improving BRD outcomes at the point of occurrence, typified by more aggressive diagnosis and treatment and using combination therapies, potentially creates vicious cycles where support of wellness outcomes decreases, animal stressors and negativity bias increase, and treatment efficacy potentially wanes. In contrast, additional focus on improving wellness outcomes can create a virtuous behavior.

EXPERIENCES USING SYSTEMS MODELING (CAUSAL LOOP DIAGRAM) FOR CONSULTING IN PRODUCTION SYSTEMS

1. Models that do not contain people and human resource management are severely limited in utility. All cattle systems are also people systems and benefit from managing as such. A significant issue in managing complex systems is emergence of new behaviors in people over time and in response to system changes. For example, caretakers will manage differently as health outcomes change, as will management. These changes can be anticipated and managed with good modeling.
2. Related to above, respect emergence in complex systems. Systems of living organisms will evolve continuously. There is no permanent fix nor permanent systems model. It is not infrequent that the structural function of a system changes without apparent changes in the component parts.
3. Models should contain the communication to include flow of, receipt of, and action on information. All systems are information systems and benefit from

managing as such. By definition, feedback loops contain information, and information that can significantly influence system behavior that is not modeled is a liability. Delays in information development and communication in complex systems are problematic and common. Often, the solution is in finding what can be communicated to whom sooner or identifying an earlier indicator to metric. In this model, the clear communication and receipt of information between cattle and people are a primary outcome modeled.

4. Models that do not recognize and help manage constraints and opportunity costing are suboptimal. A system that runs out of something it needs fails. A resource expended suboptimally is wasted.
5. Ask the causation question. Make the models causal and search for the missing component when causation is weak. The missing component might be the management insight needed or an ESB.
6. Explore the system boundaries to determine if additional systems value or leverage can be identified. An example would be managing to affect customer relationships or market access outside the existing system construct.

EXAMPLE: MANAGING FAILURE

An example might illustrate the shortcomings of the prevailing management-of-failure feeder cattle animal health mental model: When observing recent feeder cattle placements with a client, it was noted that a significant number of animals had mild quality-of-movement symptoms. When caretakers were queried, they reported a very low level of lameness with only a couple of animals treated across multiple groups. Further investigation revealed that there were underlying physical injuries resulting from maintenance issues in the processing facilities, which were repaired and resolved the quality-of-movement issues in new placements.

The individual animal observations and judgment of the caretakers were consistent with expectations. Individual lameness scores less than 1 did not meet case definition to be pulled for examination and/or treatment. However, the sheer number of mild observations was an early indicator of different potential system problems requiring immediate investigation and intervention at the system, not individual animal, level. There was no signal in the animal health metrics that any problem might be arising because animals had not yet qualified for treatment. There was nothing being measured and recorded that allowed detection.

Caretakers were obviously not in a mental model of managing overall systems outcomes unless those outcomes were the simple sum of individual failures. They were managing individual failures, not system success. Here is an example of how an approach based on evaluation, management, and metrics of individual animal failure lacked the needed sensitivity and utility to proactively manage system-wide properties before failure occurred. In this instance, the presence of mild, easily overlooked symptoms potentially had more significance than a few cases of clinical lameness. Importantly, the ability of the client to maintain market access in an environment where mobility scoring at harvest presentation is a metric used to assess animal welfare was potentially impacted.[70]

The example reveals that cattle caregivers, including veterinarians, often have mental models tuned to recognize and respond to individual failures instead of system success. An observer likely does not apply the same perspective for quality-of-movement evaluation in feeder calves used in the prepurchase examination of a new horse or view an outcome like soundness at harvest as a very complex systems output instead of a simple sum of individual outcomes. It would be hard to argue that relatively minor mechanical injuries at processing would not potentially predispose animals to other "causes" of lameness, including infectious; that pulling and treating animals for lameness might not create additional lameness in those animals or pen mates; or that increasing levels of lameness might result in increased lameness focus and more aggressive treatment of same. This is potentially creating a vicious cycle whereby lameness produces more lameness, magnified if animals are passing back through still defective facilities. In this way, by treating a symptom, we can create more of the symptom or new symptoms. Conversely, measuring and managing for a wellness behavior like quality of movement would be more likely to recognize potential issues early, diagnose key underlying factors accurately, and intervene successfully. In the example scenario, had management waited until an unacceptable incidence of nonresponsive lameness cases accrued and performed diagnostics at that time and place, it is unlikely that the predisposing, underlying cause would have been within diagnostic reach and identified. Those diagnostics might even point to several infectious causes, to which linear, intuitive sickness paradigm solutions might create new issues in the system. In the example, managing a wellness outcome and not a subsequent failure outcome was key to practicing and managing in wellness perspective.

EXPANDING WELLNESS MENTAL MODEL TO A BROADER SYSTEMS PRACTICE PHILOSOPHY

When other animal, human, and nonbiological outcomes were examined, a false dichotomous management of failure outcomes was prevalent. Failures were often symptomatic of deficiencies and interactions elsewhere in the system instead of at the point of failure. Not uncommonly, the simple, intuitive solutions to one symptom potentially created more problems through unanticipated connections between resources or ESBs. In addition, constructs and metrics for managing system success outcomes did not exist in the mental models of personnel within the systems, nor were many applicable off-the-shelf solutions for managing success outcomes available.

Fig. 9 provides an illustration of the extension of the new wellness paradigm, managing success outcome on continuous variables, into other areas often managed as dichotomous absence of failure. An example of what a small shift in mental model, rooted in a couple of a mentor's feeder calves with a few symptoms of sickness but more symptoms of wellness, can develop into. The reader can likely expand on and improve this illustration.

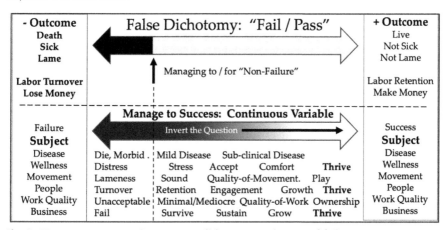

Fig. 9. Manage success continuums, not dichotomous absence of failure.

SUMMARY

In the introduction to this article, the high leverage in systems thinking of mental models and transcending paradigms, and the difficulty in recognizing and changing these cognitive biases is discussed. The difficulty extended into trying to model and teach via a personal example what a change in mental model might look like. The reader can judge the success of this article on 2 separate measures: (1) whether the new wellness mental model has utility, and (2) whether a change in mental model has been demonstrated and taught. For the purposes of this issue, the second is more important, and no introduction to systems practice would be complete without an applicable example deep in the base of the iceberg.

Any complex system measured and managed at failure breakpoints is prone to failure because it may not detect and react to early signs that the risk of failure has increased: A complex system managed on success continuums is managed further from failure. Long delays in observable system failure metrics are common. If an underlying system problem is labor, viewing it as labor instead of people may be the root of the problem, compounded by managing retention instead of employee success. Identifying other examples where managing failure is likely managing for failure is not difficult.

Holistic mental models that appreciate and leverage interconnectedness open previously unrecognized paths to improving system management and client outcomes. As mental constructs of wellness evolve and expand into new areas, and previously unrecognized connections between those areas come into focus, the ability of a veterinarian to positively influence client and animal outcomes could increase significantly. Systems practice offers an addition or alternative to the "better parts" approach of reductive science in producing continuous improvements, and possibly with fewer unanticipated and unwanted outcomes.

It is hoped that this article provides benefit to the entire audience of this issue. Those at the entry level of practice and systems thinking may only take away that stress and sickness produce similar appearance, and that wellness behavior expression can assist timely and accurate diagnosis of disease. Those further along in the professional journey might develop a more complex perspective on using wellness behaviors while remaining in disease management, production enhancement, and product-centric paradigms. It is hoped that some will see value in changing mental models into wellness perspective, pursue additional competence in system science and system modeling, and proactively use systems science to manage for positive ESBs like wellness in a new paradigm.

Better systems perspectives are needed regardless of whether we wish to avoid unintended consequences or identify new paths to desirable outcomes. A potential systems practice professional development journey might be to first undertake changing one's mental models from reductionism into wholeness perspectives using systems science tools, then redefining success along wellness spectrums instead of as the dichotomous absence of failure, then developing with clients a shared vision and metrics around those new perspectives. The author of this article believes, wholeheartedly, that emergent behaviors in complex systems hold the potential to create outbreaks of wellness and success in a new paradigm.

DISCLOSURE

T.R. Falkner is employed by Elanco Animal Health, Greenfield, Indiana, as a technical consultant. Elanco Animal Health did not provide support for nor influence this manuscript.

REFERENCES

1. Meadows D. In: Wright D, editor. Thinking in systems: a primer. London: Earth-scan; 2009.
2. Vander Ley B, Loy JD, Wollums A. Using mental models to improve understanding of cattle diseases. Vet Clin N Am Food Anim Pract 2022. In this issue.
3. Goodman M. The iceberg model. Hopkinton, MA: Innovation Associates Organizational Learning; 2002.
4. Meadows D. Leverage points: places to intervene in a system. Hartland, VT: The Sustainability Institute; 1999.
5. Kuhn T. The structure of scientific revolutions. Chicago: University of Chicago Press; 1962.
6. Fani Marvasti F, Stafford RS. From sick care to health care–reengineering prevention into the U.S. system. N Engl J Med 2012;367(10):889–91.
7. Senge P. The fifth discipline: the art and practice of the learning organization. New York: Doubleday; 2006. p. 175.
8. Rutten-Ramos SC, Simgee S, Calvo-Lorenzo MS, et al. Population-level analysis of antibiotic use and death rates in beef feedlots over ten years in three cattle-feeding regions of the United States. JAVMA 2021;259(11):1–11.
9. Vogel GJ, Bokenkroger GJ, Rutten-Ramos SC, et al. A retrospective evaluation of animal mortality in US feedlots: rate, timing and cause of death. Bovine Pract 2019;49:113–22.
10. Health. 2021. In Merriam-Webster.com. Retrieved 24 January 2021, Available at: https://www.merriam-webster.com/dictionary/health.
11. Constitution of the World Health Organization. In. Basic documents 49th edition (including amendments adopted up to 31 May 2019). Geneva: World Health Organization; 2020. p. 1.
12. Corbin CB.; Pangrazi RP. Toward a uniform definition of wellness: a commentary. President's Council on Physical Fitness and Sports 2001. Washington, DC. Research Digest 3(15); 2001-Dec:1-10.
13. Veterinarian's Oath. American Veterinary Medical Association. Retrieved 24 January 2021, from Available at: https://www.avma.org/resources-tools/avma-policies/veterinarians-oath.
14. Mellor J, BeauSoleil N. Extending the 'five domains' model for animal welfare assessment to incorporate positive welfare states. Anim Welfare 2015;24:241–53.
15. Fogsgaard KK, Rontved CM, Sorensen P, et al. Sickness behavior in dairy cow during Escherichia coli mastitis. J Dairy Sci 2012;95:630–8.
16. Mandel R, Nicol CJ, Whay HR, et al. Detection and monitoring of metritis in dairy cows using an automated grooming device. J Dairy Sci 2016;100:1–5.
17. Beaver A, Ritter C, von Keyserlingk M. The dairy cattle housing dilemma: natural behavior versus animal care. Vet Clin N Am Food Anim Pract 2019;35(1):11–27.
18. Vindevoghel TV, Fleming PA, Hyndman TH, et al. Qualitative behavioural assessment of Bos indicus cattle after surgical castration. Appl Anim Behav Sci 2019; 211:95–102.
19. Mellor DJ, Beausoleil NJ, LIttlewood KE, et al. The 2020 five domains model: including human-animal interactions in assessments of animal welfare. Animals (Basel) 2020;10(10):1870.
20. Whittum TE, Woollen NE, Perino LJ, et al. Relationships among treatment for respiratory tract disease, pulmonary lesions evident at slaughter and rate of weight gain in feedlot cattle. J Am Vet Med Assoc 1996;209:814–8.

21. Gardner BA, Dolezal HG, Bryant LK, et al. Health of finishing steers: effects on performance, carcass traits, and meat tenderness. J Anim Sci 1999;77:3168–75.
22. Bryant LK, Perino LJ, Griffin D, et al. A method for recording pulmonary lesions of beef calves at slaughter, and the association of lesions with average daily gain. Bovine Pract 1999;33(2):163–73.
23. Timsit E, Dendukuri N, Schiller I, et al. Diagnostic accuracy of clinical illness for bovine respiratory disease (BRD) diagnosis in beef cattle placed in feedlots: a systematic literature review and hierarchical Bayesian latent-class meta-analysis. Prev Vet Med 2016;135:67–73.
24. Tizard I. Sickness behavior, its mechanisms and significance. Anim Health Res Rev 2008;9(1):87–99.
25. Hart BL, Hart LA. Sickness behavior in animals: implications in health and wellness. In: Choe J, et al, editors. Encyclopedia of animal behavior. 2nd edition. Amsterdam: Academic Press; 2019. p. 171–5.
26. Wilson BK, Richards CJ, Step DL, et al. Beef species symposium: best management practices for newly weaned calves for improved health and well-being. J Anim Sci 2017;95(5):2170–82.
27. McCormick CM, Mathews IZ, Thomas C, et al. Investigations of HPA function and the enduring consequences of stressors in adolescence in animal models. Brain Cogn 2010;72(1):73–85.
28. Richeson JT. Vaccinating high risk calves against BRD. AABP 48th Proc Annu Conf 2015;48:172–5.
29. Ladewig J. Chronic intermittent stress: a model for the study of long-term stressors. In: Moberg GP, Mench JA, editors. The biology of animal stress. New York: CABI Publishing; 2000. p. 162.
30. Doyle RE, Lee C, Deiss V, et al. Measuring judgement bias and emotional reactivity in sheep following long-term exposure to unpredictable and aversive events. Physiol Behav 2011;102:503–10.
31. Baciadonna L, McElligott AG. The use of judgement bias to assess welfare in farm livestock. Anim Welfare 2015;24:81–91.
32. Lecorps B, Weary DM, von Keyserlingk MAG, et al. Pessimism and fearfulness in dairy calves. Sci Rep 2018;8:1421.
33. Destrez A, Deiss V, Leterrier C, et al. Repeated exposure to positive events induces optimistic-like judgment and enhances fearfulness in chronically stressed sheep. Appl Anim Behav Sci 2014;154:30–8.
34. Ceballos M, Sant'Anna A, Bolvin X, et al. Impact of good practices of handling training on beef cattle welfare and stockpeople attitudes and behaviors. Livestock Sci 2018;216:24–31.
35. Hemsworth PH, Coleman GJ. Human-livestock interactions: the stockperson and the productivity and welfare of intensively-farmed animals. 2nd edition. Wallingford, UK: CABI International; 2011. p. 194.
36. Hemsworth PH, Barnett JL, Coleman GJ, et al. A study of the relationships between the attitudinal and behavioural profiles of stockpeople and the level of fear of humans and the reproductive performance of commercial pigs. Appl Anim Behav Sci 1989;189(23):301–14.
37. Toaff-Rosenstein RL. The sickness response in bovine respiratory disease. Dissertation. University of California. Davis: ProQuest Dissertations Publishing; 2016.
38. Miles D. Overview of the North American beef cattle industry and the incidence of bovine respiratory disease (BRD). Anim Health Res Rev 2009;10(2):101–3.

39. White BJ, Goehl DR, Amrine DE, et al. Bayesian evaluation of clinical diagnostic test characteristics of visual observations and remote monitoring to diagnose bovine respiratory disease in beef calves. Prev Vet Med 2016;126:74–8.

40. Hazard MG. Thoughts and advice from an old cattleman. West Point, MS: Hazard Cattle Company; 2002. p. 33.

41. Wolfger B, Timsit E, White BJ, et al. A systematic review of bovine respiratory disease diagnosis focused on diagnostic confirmation, early detection, and prediction of unfavorable outcomes in feedlot cattle. Vet Clin North Am Food Anim Pract 2015;31(3):351–65.

42. Love WJ, Lehenbauer TW, Kass PH, et al. Development of a novel clinical scoring system for on-farm diagnosis of bovine respiratory disease in pre-weaned dairy calves. Peer J 2014;2e:e238.

43. Armine D. Diagnosis of bovine respiratory disease. Dissertation. Manhattan, KS: Kansas State University; 2014.

44. Napolitano F, Knierim U, Grass F, et al. Positive indicators of cattle welfare and their applicability to on-farm protocols. Ital J Anim Sci 2009;8(sup1):355–65.

45. Brambell F. Report of the technical committee to inquire into the welfare of animals kept under intensive livestock husbandry systems. London: Her Majesty's Stationary Office; 1965. p. 63–5.

46. Mellor DJ. Moving beyond the "Five Freedoms" by updating the "Five Provisions" and introducing aligned "animal welfare aims. Animals (Basel) 2016;6(10):59.

47. Foods Tyson. Tyson Foods integrating the five domains animal welfare framework across global operations. [Press release]. Springdale, AR. 2012. Available at: https://www.tysonfoods.com/news/news-releases/2021/7/tyson-foods-integrating-five-domains-animal-welfare-framework-across.

48. Verbrugghe E, Boyen F, Gaastra W, et al. The complex interplay between stress and bacterial infections in animals. Vet Microbiol 2012;155(2–4):115–27.

49. Edwards E, Cooper C. The impacts of positive psychological states on physical health: a review and theoretical framework. Social Sci Med 2020;27(12):1447–59.

50. Monat JP, Gannon TF. What is systems thinking? A review of selected literature plus recommendations. Am J Syst Sci 2015;4(1):11–26.

51. Ackoff RL. Towards a system of systems concept. Management Sci July 1971; 17(11):661–71.

52. Rethorst D. Flippin' the iceberg: a systems thinking approach to immunology and vaccination protocols in beef cow-calf systems. Proc AABP New Graduate Conf 2021;54(1):90–7.

53. O'Connor AM, Hu D, Totten SC, et al. A systematic review and network meta-analysis of bacterial and viral vaccines, administered at or near arrival at the feedlot, for control of bovine respiratory disease in beef cattle. Anim Health Res Rev 2019; 20(2):143–62.

54. Richeson JT, Falkner TR. Bovine respiratory disease vaccination: what is the effect of timing? Vet Clin N Am Food Anim Pract 2020;36(2):473–85.

55. Stokka GL, Edwards AJ, Spire MF, et al. Inflammatory response to clostridial vaccines in feedlot cattle. J Am Vet Med Assoc 1994;204(3):415–9.

56. Baccili CC, Martin CC, Decaris N, et al. Effects of 3 different commercial vaccines formulations against BVDV and BHV-1 on the Inflammatory response of Holstein heifers. Vet Sci 2019;6(3):69.

57. Tizard IR. Adverse consequences of vaccination. Vaccin Veterinarians 2021;115–30.e1.

58. Griebel PJ. BVDV vaccination in North America: risks versus benefits. Anim Health Res Rev 2015;16(1):27–32.

59. Richeson JT, Kegley EB, Gadberry MS, et al. Effects of on-arrival versus delayed clostridial or modified live respiratory vaccinations on health, performance, bovine viral diarrhea virus type I titers, and stress and immune measures of newly received beef calves. J Anim Sci 2009;87:2409–18.

60. Walz PH, Chamorro MF, Falknenberg SM, et al. Bovine viral diarrhea virus: an updated American College of Veterinary Internal Medicine consensus statement with focus on virus biology, hosts, immunosuppression, and vaccination. J Vet Intern Med 2020;34(5):1690–706.

61. Rogers KC, Miles DG, Renter DG, et al. Effects of delayed respiratory viral vaccine and/or inclusion of an immunostimulant on feedlot health, performance, and carcass merits of auction-market derived feeder heifers. Bovine Pract 2016;50(2):154–64.

62. Powledge S, Richeson J, Falkner R, et al. Clinical effects and Histophilus somni prevalence in high-risk calves administered intranasal or parenteral vaccine. Proceedings of the 102nd Conference of Research Workers in Animal Diseases 2021;218:190.

63. Snyder ER, Credille BC, Heins BD. Systematic review and meta-analysis comparing arrival versus delayed vaccination of high-risk beef cattle with 5-way modified-live viral vaccines against BHV-1, BRSV, PI3 and BVD types 1 and 2. Bovine Pract 2019;53:1–7.

64. Ives SE, Richeson JT. Review article: use of antimicrobial metaphylaxis for the control of bovine respiratory disease in high-risk cattle. Vet Clin Food Anim Pract 2015;31(3):341–50.

65. Pereira RVV, Lima S, Siler JD, et al. Ingestion of milk containing very low concentration of antimicrobials: longitudinal effect on fecal microbiota composition in preweaned calves. PLoS One 2016;11:e0147525.

66. Derakhshani H, Fehr KB, Sepehri S, et al. Invited review: microbiota of the bovine udder: contributing factors and potential implications for udder health and mastitis susceptibility. J Dairy Sci 2018;101(12):10605–25.

67. Snyder E, Credille B, et al. Prevalence of multi drug antimicrobial resistance in isolates from high-risk stocker cattle at arrival and two weeks after processing. J Anim Sci 2017;95(3):1124–31.

68. Credille B. Antimicrobial resistance in Mannheimia haemolytica: prevalence and impact. Anim Health Res Rev 2020;21(2):196–9.

69. Boyd ME, Bowers AM, Engelken TJ, et al. Feed intake response of feedlot cattle following single-dose treatment of ceftiofur crystalline free acid sterile suspension or florfenicol. Bovine Pract 2006;40(1):46–50.

70. Mijares S, Calvo-Lorenzo M, Bettis N, et al. Characterization of fed cattle mobility during the COVID-19 pandemic. Animals 2021;11(6):1749.

How Forces of a Complex Adaptive System Affect Ability to Control Bovine Respiratory Disease in Feeder Cattle

John T. Groves, DVM[a],*, Timothy J. Goldsmith, DVM, MPH[b],
Jaden M. Carlson, BS, MS[c]

KEYWORDS

- Systems thinking • Cattle • Management • Bovine respiratory disease
- Antimicrobials

KEY POINTS

- Gaining an appreciation of the forces of complex adaptive systems is key to understanding the persistent nature of bovine respiratory disease in the North American beef industry.
- Systems are capable of driving their own behavior and often produce outcomes not in alignment with individual stakeholder goals despite the rational behavior of individual participants.
- Developing shared vision regarding complex problems affecting the beef production system in North America, that takes into account the perspectives and goals of all stakeholders, is crucial to successful long-term resolution of those issues.

INTRODUCTION

The conceptualization of disease plays a powerful role in defining mental models regarding bovine respiratory disease (BRD) and can limit the ability to think effectively and profoundly about fundamental interrelationships associated with this long-standing and ever-present challenge plaguing the cattle industry. The time of the ancient Greeks and Hippocrates (c. 450—c. 380 B.C.E.) marked the first period a concept of disease was disconnected from supernatural sources such as evil spirits,

[a] Livestock Veterinary Service, 917 South Aurora/ PO Box 353, Eldon, MO 65026, USA; [b] College of Veterinary Medicine, University of Minnesota, 225 Veterinary Medical Center, 1365 Gortner Avenue, St Paul, MN 55108, USA; [c] University of Nebraska, School of Veterinary and Biomedical Sciences, Great Plains Veterinary Educational Center, 820 Road 313/ PO Box 148, Clay Center, NE 68933, USA
* Corresponding author.
E-mail address: john@livestockvetservice.com

Vet Clin Food Anim 38 (2022) 295–316
https://doi.org/10.1016/j.cvfa.2022.02.006
0749-0720/22/© 2022 Elsevier Inc. All rights reserved.
vetfood.theclinics.com

demons, and gods.[1] The utility of thinking about disease causation as an imbalance of the 4 vital humors served humanity for more than 17 centuries. Without any language or concepts beyond that of the supernatural and the 4 humors, thought and knowledge were constrained by existing mental models of disease. It was not until the Renaissance that Girolamo Fracastoro (1478–1553), an Italian physician, poet, physicist, astronomer, and pathologist, published a treatise on contagion in 1546 that a more enlightened view of disease would enter the zeitgeist.[1] Although multiple philosophies such as the miasma disease theory continued to dominate western Europe until the later nineteenth century, the groundwork had been laid for Pasteur and Koch, whose work with others established the germ theory of disease (1884).[2] Many major medical advances were made in the context provided by the germ theory of disease including the birth of the immunology discipline.[3] However, as the knowledge regarding the nature of disease continued to develop and become more complex, modern epidemiology addressed problems associated with monocausal disease theory with the advent of the multifactorial model of disease.[4] Viewing the world through the multifactorial disease model has provided the basis by which most veterinary professionals are currently educated and provides the context for how most of us think about disease. The discipline of systems thinking provides methodologies that greatly expand and redefine relationships between risk factors and disease in ways that deepen and broaden our knowledge and provide previously veiled insights.[5] Because a linear causal chain of multiple factors does not take into account complex precursors to each component of the chain, and because these may well overlap and may have further complex interactions, we propose the use of nonlinear webs of causality when thinking about the nature of bovine respiratory disease.[6] Beyond the biological and intellectual constraints of contemporary disease theory and the mental models they represent is the ability to conceptualize BRD within the context of the complex adaptive system (CAS) in which it exists. The objective of this chapter is to explore from a systems thinking perspective some of the many complex interrelationships that help us understand at a deeper level why BRD has remained the costliest disease affecting our industry in the era of modern agriculture. A foundational axiom of systems thinking based on a quote commonly attributed to W. Edwards Deming, credited with launching the Total Quality Management movement, states: "Every system is perfectly designed to get the results it gets."[7] From this context, the authors explore why beef production systems in North America so reliably produce BRD. The main outcomes of this chapter are to help give insight into a fundamental principle of systems, to more directly show that systems are capable of driving their own behavior, and to open a dialogue regarding a long-term vision to be shared among system stakeholders.

Systems used in North America to raise cattle and produce beef have characteristics consistent with CASs. Clearly made up from separate segments and components geographically spread across the continent, the system can only be completely understood when looked at as a whole so that relationships and interconnectedness between the components can be studied and considered. Similar to other CASs, the cattle industry is dynamic and in a state of constant change, dependent on continual feedback from other parts of the system, and when an intervention is made on one part of the system its effects can be traced to all parts of the system. CASs have the capacity to self-organize, reorganize, and adapt based on experience and outside pressures. The relationships and feedbacks between components of a CAS are often complex, nonlinear, and usually difficult to control and accurately predict.[8] Perhaps one of the greatest utilities of systems thinking is gaining insight into how systems can drive their own behavior and how these relationships can produce unintended consequences that are often unappreciated and overlooked by other evaluation methodologies.

Current Reality

Daniel Kim, an organizational consultant, co-founder of the Massachusetts Institute of Technology Organizational Learning Center, and founding publisher of The Systems Thinker, succinctly illuminates the need to understand current reality:

"Without a clear understanding of where we are, we have no basis for effective action."[9]

Before the 1960s, the fertile ground of the Midwest that supported corn production also dominated the cattle feeding and finishing industry; however, forward-thinking cattle feeders in the Great Plains and the High Plains regions had established themselves and were taking advantage of climatic conditions that were better suited for confinement feeding as well as cheap transportation to haul feedstuffs to the cattle.[10] During the 1960s and early 1970s there was a great expansion of feeding operations located in the Great Plains and High Plains, and infrastructure needed to support large-scale production was built. As established packing house infrastructure in the Midwest became outdated and obsolete, the packing industry expanded west and followed the migration of the cattle feeding industry. Large-scale feeding operations were advantageously positioned to leverage the introduction of new technologies into increased competitiveness through efficiencies of scale and continued growth.[10] Protocols for prevention and treatment of BRD were an integral part of this development of the cattle feeding industry. Investments made in the mitigation of the impact of BRD on the bottom line were ushered onto these large-scale intensified operations by highly trained and specialized veterinarians who were developing innovative new ways to serve these production models as "consulting" veterinarians.[10] The late 1970s brought substantial breakthroughs in the understanding of microbial interactions and their role in the pathogenesis of BRD. These insights launched the development of immunology-based and antimicrobial-based research and development that continues to this day. The first new-generation antimicrobial labeled explicitly for the treatment of BRD was approved for use in 1988 and was a strong signal from the pharmaceutical industry of its commitment to the fight against the disease, which even when viewed historically, has remained paramount over time.[11] This commitment was reaffirmed 8 years later in 1996, as the first antimicrobial was approved for what was at the time coined "metaphylactic treatment," the mass medication of a group of animals in advance of an expected outbreak of disease. Currently defined, according to the American Veterinary Medical Association (AVMA), "antimicrobial control of disease" is now synonymous language for metaphylaxis and is more precisely defined:

1. Control is the administration of an antimicrobial to an individual animal with a subclinical infection to reduce the risk of the infection becoming clinically apparent, spreading to other tissues or organs, or being transmitted to other individuals.
2. On a population basis, control is the use of antimicrobials to reduce the incidence of infectious disease in a group of animals that already has some individuals with evidence of infectious disease or evidence of infection.[12]

The year 1988 can be appreciated as a pivotal year and perhaps the beginning of the current modern era in our efforts to manage and control BRD, as it marked the first time the 3 essential components contributed to the effort:

1. the availability of professional veterinary consultative services,

2. the research and development effort for effective vaccine against microbes known to be associated with BRD, and
3. the research and development effort for antimicrobials specifically designed and approved for BRD.

The current modern era can be viewed as the era in which significant technological advances have dominated efforts to address BRD. Consequently, our examination into understanding our current reality will have a starting point of 1988.

As discussed by other investigators in this volume, the imagery of an iceberg plays a key role in thinking deeply about complex problems. Similar to icebergs, only small parts of complex problems are apparent, and for the purpose of this chapter, the problem we are most aware of is that BRD is endemic in our production systems, creating significant economic and societal impacts. Increasingly obvious to parties involved are the societal shock waves related to antimicrobial use that arise from how BRD is currently managed. Widespread bacterial pathogen resistance to antimicrobials commonly used for BRD is a very real concern shared by producers, practitioners, and the animal health industry.[13] Between 2011 and 2016, there was a significant increase in the prevalence of multidrug-resistant isolates of *Mannheimia haemolytica* and *Pasteurella multocida* associated with BRD.[14] Perhaps because our view of infectious disease is so shaped by an orientation on the importance of vaccinations, chemotherapeutic treatment, and supportive therapy, we tend to overlook the fact that animals and people have been exposed to, and have survived, the effects of disease-causing microbes through millions of years of evolutionary history.[15] In May 2015, the sixty-eighth World Health Assembly recognized the importance of the public health problem posed by antimicrobial resistance by adopting the Global Action Plan on Antimicrobial Resistance.[16] The global action plan proposes interventions to control antimicrobial resistance, including reducing the unnecessary use of antimicrobials in humans and animals. These guidelines present evidence-based recommendations and best practice statements to preserve the effectiveness of medically important antimicrobials in both human and veterinary medicine.[17]

Limits to Success—How Bovine Respiratory Disease Constrains Beef Production Systems

Despite continued improvement and effectiveness of vaccines and other technologies, BRD persists as the most economically significant disease affecting the cattle industry.[18] Analysis of a large database of feedlot closeouts containing more than 73 million head points to trends that highlight the inability of the industry as a whole to make meaningful and sustainable gains in BRD mortality losses. Respiratory death loss averaged 0.091% of monthly occupancy from 2005 through 2007, 0.097% from 2008 through 2010, and 0.127% of monthly occupancy from 2011 through 2013. (**Fig. 1**)[19] Quantifying the economic ramifications related to BRD has grown in sophistication, providing more precise understanding of the relationship between BRD and economic performance. Economic models constructed by Dennis and colleagues suggest that metaphylaxis as a BRD control tool has a value of $1.81 billion to $2.32 billion per year in producer surplus as calculated by an equilibrium displacement model.[19,20]

As beef systems evolved from local and regional models in the corn-belt to large-scale modern feeding operations that exist today, the veterinary profession and related scientific fields played integral roles in managing the impact of BRD that was in many senses co-evolving with the industry. From the systems thinking perspective, any technology introduced to beef production models that enhanced

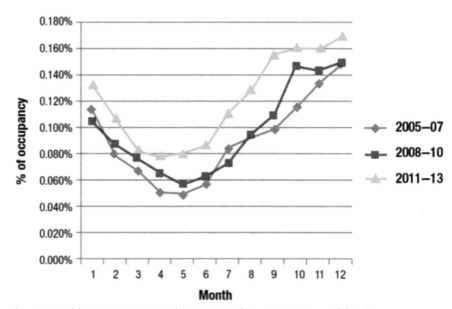

Fig. 1. Monthly respiratory mortality, expressed as a percentage of feedlot occupancy, in steers and heifers from January 1, 2005 through December 31, 2013. (*From* Vogel GJ, Bokenkroger CD, Rutten-Ramos SC, et al. A retrospective evaluation of animal mortality in US feedlots: rate, timing, and cause of death. Bov Pract (Stillwater) 2015;49:113-123; with permission.)

the ability to manage BRD became an "engine of growth." When viewing the system in the context of the archetype "limits to success," the role of expanded use of antimicrobials in the control of BRD has been a driver of growth in production units, as they are able to mitigate the constraints placed on production systems by the increasing levels of BRD that had previously been associated with production intensification. The advantages of mass medication for high-risk cattle include reduced sickness rate, potential to reduce mortality, less labor required, and improved gains.[21]

Perhaps the best example of how an antimicrobial became an "engine of growth" in cattle production systems is the approval of an antimicrobial with label approval for control of BRD in 1996.[11] Operations previously constrained by their ability to manage BRD on their operations could implement metaphylaxis and have an opportunity for growth and capturing economies of scale previously out of their reach. Just as profound as the ability of metaphylaxis to mitigate BRD during the arrival phase was the fact that the effect was nearly immediate and did not require a protracted delay in systems feedback that was associated with other technologies and management approaches. The more effective the tactic of metaphylaxis became and the more immediate the feedback, the more it enhanced the operations' ability to acquire and manage cattle and increase the potential to be profitable, thereby fueling growth. In the language of systems thinking, the operations had entered into a virtuous reinforcing loop in which metaphylaxis mitigated the impact of BRD, which led to operational growth with more feeder calf purchases, which allowed the operations to increase revenues and marketplace competitiveness. Operations remained in this virtuous reinforcing loop as long as the metaphylactic drug was effective and could control BRD levels to rates acceptable in an economic cost to benefit analysis (**Fig. 2**).

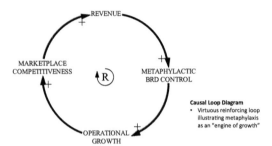

Fig. 2. Reinforcing feedback loop.

Interestingly, the growth fueled by the application of this technology was eventually governed by other powerful systems-level interactions and forces at play. Microbial populations that play necessary roles in the pathogenesis of BRD continued down an evolutionary path that was now influenced by mass use of antimicrobials. After a significant delay, the efficacy of compounds was reduced, and BRD rates increased to levels at which they limited the growth and revenue generating ability of the production model, once again becoming a constraint.[22] In systems language, the process in which a limiting variable reemerges in a system is the product of a balancing loop that is part of the natural structure providing equilibrium. In the case at hand, we can view the balancing process in which microbial communities achieve homeostasis with hosts. When viewed together with the "engine of growth," we can better understand the relationship between the development of antimicrobial resistance and the utility of metaphylaxis. The system will behave according to which feedback loop is dominant at that particular point in time (**Box 1, Fig. 3**).

Development of compound resistance over time illustrates an important concept in systems thinking. Established systems, especially those containing a biological component, are very resistant to long-term change and often "push back" in an effort to regain system homeostasis.[23] Because the effects of metaphylaxis have driven such profound change in production models, the industry has invested tremendous research and development resources into recapturing the "engine of growth" that can exist while antimicrobial compounds retain their efficacy. What started as a single approval in 1996 has progressed over time into a trend in which antimicrobial development and approvals for control has paralleled approvals for treatment (**Fig. 4**).

Box 1
Dominance

Dominance is an important concept in systems thinking. Shifting dominance of feedback loops occurs when one loop dominates another, and it has a stronger impact on behavior. Systems usually have several competing feedback loops operating at the same time, so the loops that dominate the system at any point in time will drive behavior. When metaphylaxis was introduced, antimicrobial resistance was low, and the reinforcing loop became an engine of growth. But antimicrobial resistance has increased over time weakening that reinforcing loop. Eventually, the balancing loop representing the development of resistance will be equal in strength to the growth loop, and the system will be in dynamic equilibrium.

Adapted from Meadows D. *Thinking in Systems A Primer.* London, UK: Earthscan; 2009; with permission.

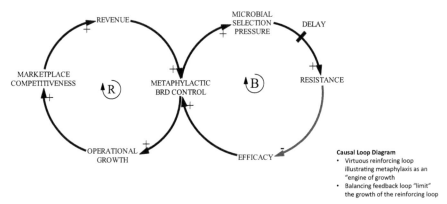

Fig. 3. Limits to success.

During the past 25 years the pharmaceutical industry has successfully developed and launched new antimicrobial compounds that have worked in addressing the emergence of microbial resistance to existing approved drugs.[11] From the perspective of new compound development, we can now clearly identify a new constraint or limiting variable in the system. Can new antimicrobials be developed at a rate that exceeds the rate at which current antimicrobials lose their efficacy due to resistance, and if they can be developed, are there broader global systems concerns that will limit our access to them (**Fig. 5**)?

An important consideration to understanding the role of the "limits to growth" archetype in a system is comprehending that this structure may have existed for some time during which the constraint or limit has been addressed to some extent through innovation. Previous successful efforts to manage constraints produce "boom" times allowing opportunity for growth. Over time, the resources devoted to and effort needed to drive that level of innovation become more and more extensive and consume more and more resources.[23] In reality, limitless growth is not possible, and innovative solutions to constraints become more and more cumbersome and difficult over time. In an effort to gain insight into the resources being

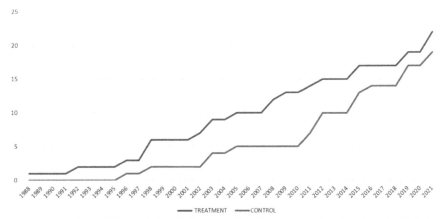

Fig. 4. Cummulative FDA antimicrobial approvals-BRD treatment label and control label.

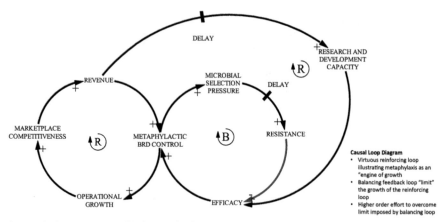

Fig. 5. Limits to success—higher order limit.

devoted to finding technology to mitigate the impact of BRD since 1988, we queried scientific literature databases using Google Scholar by year for quantity of results from 1988 through 2020 as a means of semiquantifying the amount of scientific effort being devoted toward BRD by year and compared that with an equivalent approach for an index disease (diarrhea, scours) of beef cattle. Understanding trends over time is key in understanding important systems structures driving the behavior in the system. Often, the cognitive processes required to understand complex interconnections in systems require access and insight into variables and trends not traditionally recorded, tracked, or monitored. When dependable data regarding variables of interest do not exist, systems thinkers often hypothetically test or sample the relationships of associated variables. Admittedly unscientific, the methodology of these "thought experiments" allow the use of surrogate "soft" variables viewed over time to gain insight into trends and patterns existing in the system (**Fig. 6, Table 1**).

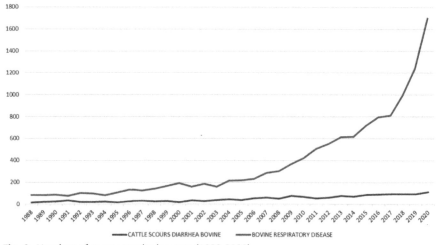

Fig. 6. Number of query results by year (1988-2020).

Table 1
Number of query results by year

Year	"Cattle" "Scours" "Diarrhea" "Bovine"	"Bovine Respiratory Disease"
1988	17	85
1989	21	85
1990	24	86
1991	35	77
1992	21	104
1993	22	100
1994	25	85
1995	19	110
1996	28	135
1997	33	126
1998	27	142
1999	28	169
2000	19	194
2001	35	162
2002	29	186
2003	39	160
2004	45	215
2005	37	219
2006	53	233
2007	61	288
2008	52	304
2009	76	368
2010	69	422
2011	54	508
2012	61	552
2013	77	614
2014	71	618
2015	88	719
2016	90	795
2017	92	811
2018	94	1000
2019	92	1240
2020	112	1700

Query results by year comparing "Bovine Respiratory Disease" with a combination of terms related to enteric disease.
Data from Google Scholar.

From the perspective of beef production, introduction of new antimicrobial technologies can be seen as novel and innovative solutions addressing the limits that BRD placed on the industry. Each new compound or approved use led to "boom" times and fueled growth. This effectively describes the role of antimicrobials in the evolution of the beef industry. As expected, microbial communities have coevolved with the system and adapted to the increased antimicrobial pressure.[22]

Antimicrobial use in beef production systems is currently an issue of great concern. From a narrow systems view, it is not sustainable in the long-term, and from a broader systems view, societal pressures on the food production system concerning implications to human health continue to indicate that future reliance on this technology will be more highly regulated, monitored, and possibly discontinued.[24] Consumer and societal preferences and demands balanced against production efficiency and global food supply will become increasingly important features in the algorithm.

Systems dynamics modelers observe 2 different patterns of behavior when a system that has depended on removing limits to drive growth is unable to innovate further improvements. First, instead of having booms the system could plateau and reach a state of equilibrium requiring massive effort to introduce new technology just to maintain current performance. Second, and less desirably, after overshooting its natural constraints, the system collapses into what systems modelers call the phenomenon of "overshoot and collapse."[23] Whether, as a beef system, we are approaching the "tipping point" or the threshold at which the system changes radically and seeks a new point of equilibrium is a question worth consideration. The trend represented by the exponential growth of scientific publications associated with BRD suggest we could be approaching a tipping point. From the viewpoint of Meadows and colleagues, effectively, as an industry we can either choose at what limit we can be sustainable or at some point reach the imposed limit of the system, at which time collapse is unavoidable.[25]

As systems evolve and struggle to find solutions that require high levels of effort, they become susceptible to higher level constraint with much farther-reaching implications, such as loss of system-wide support and shared vision (**Box 2— hierarchy**).

The "limits to success" archetype should not be used as a tool when a growth-limiting constraint is discovered, rather it is most impactful to understand how the cumulative effects of removing constraints have led to our current reality and how continual removal of those constraints could lead to future problems.[9]

Box 2
Hierarchy

Self-organization often generates hierarchies of subsystems as they become increasingly complex. Even though in some respects a commercial cow-calf operation can seem infinitely complex, it can also be viewed as part of a larger system that supplies feeder cattle to feeding sector and when viewed with the feeding sector, becomes a system nested in a larger cattle industry system that provides finished cattle to the packing/processing industry, which in turn can be seen as a subsystem of the global food supply system. This arrangement of systems and subsystems is called a hierarchy.

If subsystems regulate and maintain themselves and serve the needs of the larger system, while the larger system coordinates and enhances the functioning of the subsystems, a stable, resilient, and efficient structure results. The original purpose of hierarchy is to always help its originating subsystems do their jobs better; although, when a subsystem's goal dominates at the expense of the total system's goals, the resulting behavior is called "suboptimization," and just as damaging as suboptimization is the problem of too much central control.

Adapted from Meadows D. *Thinking in Systems A Primer.* London, UK: Earthscan; 2009; with permission.

Leverage in the "limits to growth" scenario lies in its early stages, while you still have the time and resources to take action. Look for other potential drivers of growth rather than over-relying on a single constraint.[23]

Fixes that Backfire—the Story of Unintended Consequences

Addressing the impact of BRD in the North American beef production chain is an important role for all participants in the system; however, the perception that BRD is the central problem rather than a symptomatic manifestation of more fundamental causalities leads to implementations of solutions without considerations for potential long-term unintended consequences. Causal loop diagrams (CLDs) are an essential tool of the systems thinking language that allow us to see and contemplate the nature of how parts of a system are connected in a real-time dynamic way.[26] CLDs communicate in a way that help make more central observations possible. Often the first profound observation systems thinkers make is that the "event" or "problem" that initially drove them to use the thought-methodology is not the root problem at all, but merely a symptom of deeper fundamental problems. From the position of a systems thinker, it can be informative to think about BRD more precisely as a symptom arising from all the unintended consequences that result from all the rationally bound decisions made elsewhere in system. A common theme found in systems thinking methodologies is that the problems of today arise from solutions of the past.[27] Decision-making in the absence of an appreciation or understanding of its systems-wide ramifications results in the predictably constant emergence of unintended consequences. Decisions should be and are driven by rational thought; however, when thought processes only consider a single position in a system rather than considering the whole system, they are "bounded" and often produce deleterious side effects for the rest of the system. The concept of bounded rationality was first described by Nobel Prize–winning American economist Herbert Simon.[28] Simon's work in behavioral economics provides insights into understanding why members of an economy make decisions based on individual benefits rather than benefits to the society as a whole. The highly diverse and segmented nature of the beef production industry in North America amplifies the potential of bounded rationality affecting the system. The underlying structure of our capitalistic economy further motivates individuals within the different parts of the system to make decisions not based on what is best for the system in the long term, but what is most beneficial to them and the part of the system in which the individual is involved.

The archetype "fixes that backfire" is a useful and powerful tool that informs systems level understanding of why decisions made to "fix" problems afflicting a local part of a system can "backfire" and have unforeseen harmful implications in other parts of the system. The core principle of the archetype is that all decisions have both short-term and long-term consequences, and more often than not, they are utterly opposed.[23]

One of the most profound and powerful mental models in American and global agriculture is the quest for increases in production efficiency. This nearly universal and fundamental mental model has played a primary role, not only in formation of political and regulatory policy but also in how we have taught, trained, and educated generations of agriculturalists and even, to some extent, affected our culture. The principle of managing and driving down unit cost of production is well understood and demonstrated in the beef production system as well; however, most people involved in those efforts rarely consider the unintended costs associated with drive for efficiency.

An often-used tactic to drive efficiency is to capture economies of scale. As operations grow, they gain numerous economies such as the ability to gain discounts on input purchases, achieve premiums on output sale, and spread costs over more units, thereby lowering investment per unit. This archetype usually begins when a performance metric is outside an unacceptable threshold. In production agriculture, the impetus is often that the unit cost of production is viewed as too high; thus, management looks for opportunities to address the situation by increasing the number of units purchased to provide a balancing feedback process to correct the metric back to less than the acceptable threshold (**Fig. 7**).

Although the benefits of economies of scale are undeniable as a driver of growth across nearly all economic systems and as an effort to manage unit cost of production, a systems view behooves us to consider the ramifications and consequences, both intentional and unintentional, of the decision to scale up operations. The increase in the number of calves purchased can and does have many unintended consequences, from stretched human and infrastructure resources to the change in the risk and dynamics of microbial pathogens. The latter will be considered in this example, although the reader is encouraged to think deeply about all the potential unintended consequences associated with this scenario.

Increases in the number of calves entering an operation changes the dynamics of microbial pathogens and risk probabilities associated with those microbes. At some tipping point this leads to increased rates of BRD, thereby leading to incremental increases in unit cost of production. Understanding the structure of this archetype provides insight into and partially explains a commonly observed behavior of cattle production systems: they will tolerate BRD rates up to the point it affects unit cost of production greater than a threshold level linked to profitability. Once the threshold of tolerance for BRD is exceeded, policy makers within the system feel pressure to take actions to correct the trend and often use tactics that have been successful solutions in the past. In the example at hand, the system would respond by purchasing even more calves to capture even larger economies of scale in an effort to balance the unit cost problem. Understanding the structure that drives the behavior in systems illustrates that, in most complex situations, rational decisions are being made locally that produce detrimental unintended consequences at a global system level (**Fig. 8**).

Shifting the Burden—the Story of Addiction

"Limits to growth" and "fixes that backfire" archetypes play profound roles of enlightenment in our understanding of systems level forces at play in our efforts to mitigate the impact of BRD in our production models. These archetypes help explain why many of our efforts, although perhaps successful in the short term, usually fail in the long term and quite often become sources of emerging problems of the future. "Shifting the burden" archetype, in addition to examining the implications of short-term

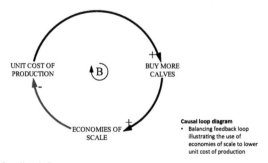

Fig. 7. Balancing feedback loop.

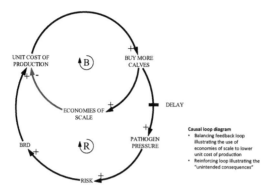

Fig. 8. Fixes that backfire.

solutions, also examines how they can affect our ability to address fundamental root causal factors in a sustainable way. In more precise systems language, this archetype helps us think deeply about how to address symptoms in a system and affects our ability to address the fundamental causes leading to the expression of that symptom. Certainly, knowledge regarding the role of the myriad of contributing and necessary causal risk factors associated in BRD's web of causality has grown exponentially. Unfortunately, knowledge regarding fundamental causation mechanisms remains extremely difficult to leverage into impactful long-term interventions.

"Shifting the burden" starts with an effort to "fix" a symptom associated with underlying systemic problems. In our example for this chapter, it begins with an effort to mitigate problems associated with BRD in a way that produces quickly observable results that are effective in the short term at alleviating the symptom. As previously discussed, a common tactic used to immediately mitigate the impact of BRD is the application of metaphylactic antimicrobials in an effort to create a balancing feedback loop that alleviates the symptom (**Fig. 9**).

However, forces also exist at a systems level to address the fundamental factors leading to the development of BRD in the first place. Interventions that address causation at a root level are often more difficult to implement and generally take an extended amount of time before an impact can be measured. Depending on the frame of reference, variables such as genetic resistance to disease, biocontainment efforts that minimize pathogen exposure and pathogen amplification, stress mitigation efforts, immunologic efforts that build disease resistance, husbandry efforts that promote natural behaviors, and nutritional support of homeostasis, as well as countless other variables are associated with addressing fundamental issues in the web of causation. In

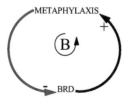

Fig. 9. Balancing feedback loop.

the context of this example, managing these root cause issues can be seen as fundamental long-term solutions in the causal loop diagram (**Fig. 10**).

In an ideal world, policy makers would take a balanced and prudent approach to how many resources get devoted to each balancing loop. In the long-term, it is logical to invest in fundamental solutions that reduce or eliminate the need for short-term fixes. However, because of delays, the balancing loop associated with fundamental solutions is slow at producing results. This difference in feedback delays lies at the core of the unintended consequences associated with this archetype—the loop of addiction. In times of crisis, such as a difficult-to-manage BRD outbreak, management learns and is rewarded for reacting in ways that produce quick, tangible results in scenarios known as "crisis heroism."[23] Heroic efforts made over time are recognized as important accomplishments, and responsible individuals are often promoted. Meanwhile, the need to address long-term root causes becomes increasingly more critical; however, efforts made in those arenas often go unrecognized and unrewarded even when gains are made. Over time, the system becomes more and more dependent on implementers of short-term fixes and reduces investments in long-term solutions that are slow to pay off (**Box 3**).

The unintended consequence is the "loop of addiction," which creates dependence on "heroes" implementing short-term symptomatic fixes at the cost of progress in fundamental root cause solutions. Over time, repeated systematic rewards for short-term solutions for heroes leads operations to decrease investments aimed at addressing long-term fundamental cures, leaving them only motivated to address symptoms rather than root causes. The extended turnaround times associated with long-term solutions can work to disincentivize investments in those efforts. More strikingly apparent to the systems perspective is the lack of reward feedback mechanisms for efforts that are challenging to execute and have long time horizons. In the words of systems dynamists Repenning and Sterman, "Nobody ever gets credit for fixing problems that never happened"[29](**Fig. 11**).

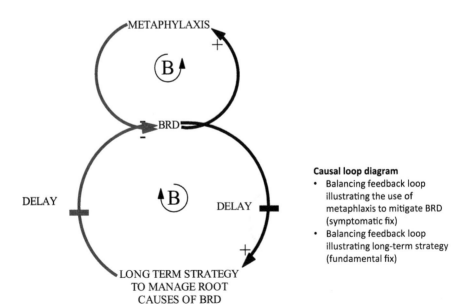

Fig. 10. Balancing symptomatic fix loop with balancing fundamental fix loop.

Box 3
Self-organization

The ability of a system to develop its own increasingly complex structure is called "self-organization." This characteristic drives a system's ability to learn, diversify, become more complex, and evolve.

Self-organization fuels innovation, creativity, and heterogeneity. The process requires freedom of thought and experimentation, which may be threatening to existing power structures.

Systems theorists used to think that self-organization was such a complex property of systems that it could never be understood. New discoveries, however, suggest that just a few simple organizing principles can lead to widely diverse self-organizing structures.

Adapted from Meadows D. *Thinking in Systems A Primer.* London, UK: Earthscan; 2009; with permission.

Tragedy of the Commons—the Story of Shared Limited Resources

A "commons" is a resource shared and used by a group. The term was initially used to describe common land ownership in small European towns. These commons were used to support grazing livestock owned within the community.[30] Garrett Hardin, an American ecologist, first popularized the term "Tragedy of the Commons" in his 1968 paper warning of overpopulation.[31] Commons has come to mean all the resources accessible to members of a group. Some noteworthy qualities of resource commons are that they are limited in their amount at any point in time but have the ability to renew and regenerate when they are used in a way that allows them to restore. Tragedy occurs when their ability to regenerate is overwhelmed and damaged. Perhaps the most relatable example of a commons is a shared pasture of finite carrying capacity. Any individual rancher that adds more cattle to that pasture in an effort to benefit individually in the short term endangers the entire community through the risk of overgrazing in the long term. As the forage is overgrazed, the plants develop less extensive root systems that support less plant growth and consequently are

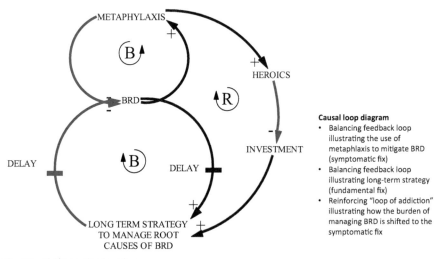

Fig. 11. Shifting the burden.

less efficient at preventing soil erosion. Over time, plant growth is compromised, erosion becomes problematic, and the system crashes because the ability of the commons to regenerate was compromised.

For the purposes of this chapter, the common resource of interest is the pharmacologic resource encompassing all the antimicrobial products approved for the treatment and control of BRD. As of the writing of this chapter, that resource contains 23 approvals with a treatment claim and 21 approvals for a control claim[11] (Table 2).

Because antimicrobials play such a key role in BRD mitigation in the industry today, they can be seen as a resource of critical importance. How we manage this resource is a point of high leverage in the system in which we produce beef, but also in the more global systems perspectives such as human health and environmental science. Thinking about these antimicrobials as a commons helps us understand the fragile balance associated with how it should be managed.

In the United States, the Food and Drug Administration (FDA) has authority over the approval, labeling, and use of antimicrobials under the Federal Food, Drug, and Cosmetic Act. Moreover, the FDA Center for Veterinary Medicine, guided policy through the Animal Medicinal Drug Use Clarification Act of 1994 (AMDUCA), defines and permits veterinarians to prescribe extralabel uses of certain approved new animal drugs and approved human drugs for animals under certain conditions. In addition, clearer guidelines regarding the definition of the veterinarian-client-patient relationship at the state level through interpretation and changes made to respective practice acts have also affected policy regarding antimicrobials. More recently, through the use of the FDA guidance process, antimicrobial use policy has been further regulated and guided from a federal level. It may be premature to know if increases in regulatory pressure regarding antimicrobials have been successful in protecting the common resource of antimicrobials from being damaged. It may be possible that users of antimicrobials at a local level feel a sense of endorsement and justification for their individual use decisions based on the level of governmental oversight and feel empowered, as long as they remain in compliance with federal and state regulations. From a broader systems perspective, an improved algorithm for guiding use policy at a local level would be to focus on awareness and accountability of how the use decisions affect the common resource. At a systems level, there is tremendous leverage in antimicrobial use policy at a local level because it can drive selection pressure for resistance in ways that damage the common resource, even when the antimicrobials are used in approved ways. Approval for metaphylactic use has been incorrectly interpreted by some to mean that the product can be used in that role in all situations without regard to long-term unintended consequences. This being the case, certain players within the system, whether intentional or not, can and do take advantage of this and profit by using resources belonging to the commons in a way that deteriorates its value to the rest of the system. Recent efforts falling under the titles "Antimicrobial Stewardship" and "Judicious Drug Use" can be seen as attempts to outline key elements surrounding antimicrobial use in different settings, both human and animal, in an effort to protect this common resource.

In the language of systems thinking, we can envision and diagram a system in which 2 operations elect to use metaphylaxis in somewhat different ways: blanket use on all incoming cattle and strategic use on groups identified most at risk for BRD. Both operations attempt to build virtuous reinforcing feedback loops in which metaphylaxis improves BRD control, thereby driving the increase in the use of the policy (Fig. 12).

Both operations contribute to the total antimicrobial used system wide, but the level at which the operation using the blanket use policy contributes is much greater than the operation using strategic application (Fig. 13).

Table 2
Antimicrobial approvals for bovine respiratory disease from 1988 to 2021

Trade Name	Active Compound	Year of Approval—BRD Treatment	Year of Approval—BRD Control
Naxcel	Ceftiofur sodium	1988	NA
Micotil 300	Tilmicosin phosphate	1922	1996
Nuflor	Florfenicol	1996	1998
Baytril	Enrofloxacin	1998	2012
Excenel	Ceftiofur hydrochloride	1998	NA
Adspec	Spectinomycin sulfate Tetrahydrate	1998	NA
Advocin	Danofloxacin	2002	2011
Tetradure 300/ Noromycin 300 LA	Oxytetracycline dihydrate	2003	2003
Excede	Ceftiofur crystalline-free acid	2003	2003
Draxxin	Tulathromycin	2005	2005
NuflorGOLD	Florfenicol	2008	NA
EXCENEL RTU EZ	Ceftiofur hydrochloride	2008	NA
Resflor Gold	Florfenicol and flunixin meglumine	2009	NA
Zactran	Gamithromycin	2011	2011
Zuprevo	Tildipirosin	2012	2012
Loncor	Florfenicol	2015	2015
Norfenicol	Florfenicol	2015	2015
Enroflox	Enrofloxacin	2013	2015
Enromed	Enrofloxacin	2019	2019
Cefenil	Ceftiofur hydrochloride	2019	NA
Draxxin	Ketoprofen tulathromycin	2021	NA
MACROSYN	Tulathromycin	2021	2021
Increxxa	Tulathromycin	2021	2021
Pulmotil 90	Tilmicosin phosphate	NA	2011
Pulmotil 90 and Rumensin 90	Monensin and tilmicosin phosphate	NA	2012
Tilmovet 90	Tilmicosin phosphate	NA	2015
Tilmovet 90 and Rumensin 90	Monensin and tilmicosin phosphate	NA	2016
Tilmovet and Monovet	Monensin and tilmicosin phosphate	NA	2019
Pulmotil and Monovet	Monensin and tilmicosin phosphate	NA	2019

Antimicrobial approvals for BRD by year for treatment and control.
Data from Animal Drugs @ FDA.

Causal loop diagram
- Reinforcing feedback loops illustrating the use of two different policies to use metaphylaxis to mitigate BRD

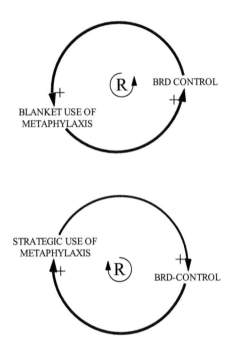

Fig. 12. Reinforcing feedback loops.

Causal loop diagram
- Reinforcing feedback loops illustrating the use of two different policies to use metaphylaxis to mitigate BRD
- Contribution to total antimicrobial use is dependent of use policy of operation

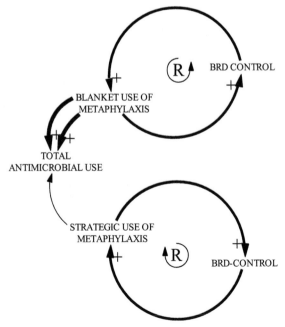

Fig. 13. Reinforcing feedback loops.

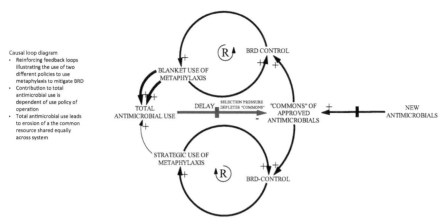

Fig. 14. Tragedy of the commons.

As discussed in "limits to growth," antimicrobials have many consequences, of which the most relevant for this example is the selection for resistance to antimicrobial compounds that occurs over time (**Fig. 14**).

In the developed archetype discussed earlier, it is apparent that inattention and damage to the commons can be tolerated by a system up to a tipping point. As long as the commons has the ability to regenerate (novel and effective antimicrobials enter the marketplace), the system remains in equilibrium. It is only when the rate at which microbes become resistant exceeds the rate at which new compounds are developed and marketed that we become aware of the instability in the system.[32]

The "tragedy to the commons" archetype highlights inequities that can exist in systems. The part of the system most responsible for overwhelming the capacity of the commons reaps the benefits singularly, if only in the short term. However, all players in the system suffer the consequences, even those that did not contribute to the demise of the shared resource. The ramifications of these inequities are further amplified in market-driven economies where competitive advantage is often linked to the ability to draw maximum benefits from shared resources. The situation in which operations most responsible for damaging the commons are at a competitive advantage in the short term, although somewhat perverse, often sets into motion another familiar systems archetype known as "success to the successful," which can further drive their competitive advantage in the marketplace.

Depletion of a common shared resource is a recurring theme across many complex problems. When a player or policy maker in the system becomes aware of the potential or actual deterioration of the shared common resource, a call to action is initiated. Most intuitive is to increase the rate at which the commons can regenerate. In the example at hand, that would mean ramping up resources devoted to a research and development pipeline for the creation of novel and effective antimicrobial compounds that could restore the ability of the commons to regenerate. However, less intuitive and perhaps more impactful is to slow the rate in which the resource is depleted and damaged through using more strategic antimicrobial use policy that extends the useful life of compounds currently in the shared resource and concentrates on the development of root cause solutions that eliminate or abate the needs for antimicrobials in the first place.

Box 4
Resilience

Resilience is the measure of a system's ability to adapt, survive, and persist over time. The opposite of resilience is inflexibility, brittleness, and fragility. Resilience is derived from a utilizing complex structure of feedback loops that can work in multiple ways to restore a system to equilibrium after serious disturbances. Although a single balancing loop can bring a system back to its desired equilibrium, true resilience is provided by many such loops operating in different ways and on different time scales.

Resilience should not be confused with being static or constant over time. Short-term oscillations, cyclical outbreaks, and long cycles of growth and retraction may be normal.

Resilience is usually not understood or appreciated without the whole-system view and is sometimes sacrificed for efficiency, productivity, security, or some other system property.

Adapted from Meadows D. *Thinking in Systems A Primer.* London, UK: Earthscan; 2009; with permission.

SUMMARY

One of the main outcomes of this chapter is to help give insight into fundamental principles of systems, in order to more directly show that systems are capable of driving their own behavior. Even when all players in a system behave in rational and scientifically based ways, the system still exerts a force of which most of us are unaware. Deep understanding of these forces lies in understanding the nature and structure of interrelationships between variables in the system, not just a deep understanding of the variables.

Another outcome is to open a dialogue regarding a long-term vision to be shared among system stakeholders. Within the discipline of systems thinking, creative tension can be generated as a tool to move toward change. In order to have creative tension or pressure to change, we need to establish a shared vision that is based on the current reality of where we are at today and a clear idea of what we wish to achieve.[9] If we accept the current reality in our case example outlined earlier for BRD in feeder cattle, the next step in establishing the creative tension is establishing a shared vision. For a CAS such as the cattle production system in North America, establishing a shared vision is a difficult task. It starts with establishing a personal vision for oneself and the development of stakeholders and clarifying the current reality with those stakeholders. Then a shared vision that takes into account the perspectives and goals of all the stakeholders can be established. Although one can envision this at a local level, or with a single producer, as we expand to multiple producers or a larger geographic area, we can see how the diversity and capitalistic nature of a segmented cattle production system can struggle to establish a shared vision. As we, as a production system, establish a shared vision, we can use the resulting tension on where we are and where we want to be to drive change toward the established goals. Tension, by its nature, seeks resolution, and the most beneficial way to resolve the tension that is our current reality is to move closer to what we really want, that being our shared vision. Paradoxically, it is important to point out that creative tension in systems battling longstanding problems of a complex nature is often resolved perniciously and stealthily over time in a much less beneficial way, lowering of the goals that were developed as a shared vision (**Box 4**).

Systems thinking approaches are tools that can be used to better articulate and ultimately understand the interrelationships within the CAS that is the cattle production system in North America, ultimately driving us to the development of solutions that address the root causes of problems rather than focusing solely on the symptom resulting from the present system.

DISCLOSURE

J.T. Groves has received honoraria to provide education on the topic of Systems Thinking to veterinarians. The other authors have nothing to disclose.

REFERENCES

1. Veith I. Historical reflections on the changing concepts of disease. Calif Med 1969;110(6):501–6.
2. Black GV. The formation of Poisons by Micro-organisms: a biological Study of the germ theory of disease. Philadelphia: P. Blakiston, Son & Co; 1884.
3. Kaufmann SHE, Winau F. From bacteriology to immunology: the dualism of specificity. Nat Immunol 2005;6(11):1063–6.
4. Broadbent A. Causation and models of disease in epidemiology. Stud Hist Philos Biol Biomed Sci 2009;40(4):302–11.
5. Hulme A, Finch CF. From monocausality to systems thinking: a complementary and alternative conceptual approach for better understanding the development and prevention of sports injury. Inj Epidemiol 2015;2(1):1–12.
6. Ventriglio A, Bellomo A, Bhugra D. Web of causation and its implications for epidemiological research. Int J Soc Psychiatry 2016;62(1):3–4.
7. Deming WE. Every system is perfectly designed to get the results it gets. The W.Edwards Deming Institute. Available at. https://deming.org/quotes/10141/. Accessed September 27, 2021.
8. Agyepong IA, Kodua A, Adjei S, et al. When 'solutions of yesterday become problems of today': crisis-ridden decision making in a complex adaptive system (CAS)—the Additional Duty Hours Allowance in Ghana. Health Policy Plan 2012;27(suppl_4):iv20–31.
9. Kim DH, Mullen E. The spirit of the learning organization. Syst Thinker 1993; 4(4):1–3.
10. Smith RA, Step DL, Woolums AR. Bovine respiratory disease: looking back and looking forward, what do we see? veterinary clinics. Vet Clin North Am Food Anim Pract 2020;36(2):239–51.
11. Food and Drug Administration. Summary report on antimicrobials Sold or Distributed for Use in food-producing animals 2019.
12. American Veterinary Medical Association. AVMA definitions of antimicrobial use for treatment, control, and prevention. AVMA Policies. Available at https://www.avma.org/resources-tools/avma-policies/avma-definitions-antimicrobial-use-treatment-control-and-prevention. Accessed September 27, 2021.
13. DeDonder KD, Apley MD. A literature review of antimicrobial resistance in pathogens associated with bovine respiratory disease. Anim Health Res Rev 2015; 16(2):125–34.
14. Klima CL, Holman DB, Cook SR, et al. Multidrug resistance in Pasteurellaceae associated with bovine respiratory disease mortalities in North America from 2011 to 2016. Front Microbiol 2020;11:1–21.
15. Hart BL. Animal behavior and the fever response: theoretical considerations. J Am Vet Med Assoc 1985;187(10):998–1001.
16. WHO Library Cataloguing-in-Publication Data Global Action Plan on Antimicrobial Resistance. I.World Health Organization. ISBN 978 92 4 150976 3 Subject headings are available from WHO institutional repository © World Health Organization

2015 All rights reserved. Publications of the World Health Organization are available on the WHO web site (www.who.int) or can be purchased from WHO Press, World Health Organization, 20 Avenue Appia, 1211 Geneva 27, Switzerland.

17. World Health Organization. (2017). WHO guidelines on use of medically important antimicrobials in food-producing animals: web annex A: evidence base. World Health Organization. https://apps.who.int/iris/handle/10665/259241. License: CC BY-NC-SA 3.0 IGO.

18. Peel DS. The effect of market forces on bovine respiratory disease. Vet Clin North Am Food Anim Pract 2020;36(2):497–508.

19. Vogel GJ, Bokenkroger CD, Rutten-Ramos SC, et al. A retrospective evaluation of animal mortality in US feedlots. Bovine Pract 2015;113–23.

20. Dennis EJ, Schroeder TC, Renter DG, et al. Value of arrival metaphylaxis in US cattle industry. J Agric Resour Econ 2018;43(2):233–50.

21. Smith RA. Health considerations for Stocker and feeder cattle. Academy of Veterinary Consultants Conference; 1994.

22. Snyder ER, Alvarez-Narvaez S, Credille BC. Genetic characterization of susceptible and multi-drug resistant Mannheimia haemolytica isolated from high-risk stocker calves prior to and after antimicrobial metaphylaxis. Vet Microbiol 2019; 235:110–7.

23. Senge PM. The fifth discipline fieldbook: Strategies and tools for building a learning organization. Currency; 1994.

24. Kirchhelle C. Pharming animals: a global history of antibiotics in food production (1935–2017). Palgrave Commun 2018;4(1):1–13.

25. Meadows DH, Meadows DL, Randers J, et al. The limits to growth: a report for the culb of rome's project on the predicament of mankind. New American Library; 1972.

26. Goodman M. Systems thinking: What, why, when, where, and how. Syst Thinker 1997;8(2):6–7.

27. Forrester JW. World dynamics. Wright-Allen Press; 1971.

28. Simon HA. Bounded rationality. Utility and probability. Springer; 1990. p. 15–8.

29. Repenning NP, Sterman JD. Nobody ever gets credit for fixing problems that never happened: creating and sustaining process improvement. Calif Manag Rev 2001;43(4):64–88.

30. Lloyd WF. Two lectures on the checks to population. JH Parker; 1833.

31. Garrett H. The tragedy of the commons. Science 1968;162:1243–8.

32. Lubbers BV, Hanzlicek GA. Antimicrobial multidrug resistance and coresistance patterns of Mannheimia haemolytica isolated from bovine respiratory disease cases—a three-year (2009–2011) retrospective analysis. J Vet Diagn Invest 2013;25(3):413–7.

Current Reality of Beef Cattle Veterinary Practice in North America

A Systems Thinking Perspective

Dale M. Grotelueschen, DVM, MS[a],*, Rebecca A. Funk, DVM, MS[b],
John T. Groves, DVM[c], Timothy J. Goldsmith, DVM, MPH, DACVPM[d],
Brian Vander Ley, DVM, PhD[b]

KEYWORDS

- Veterinarian • Practice • System • Systems thinking • Beef • Cattle • Beef cattle
- Veterinary profession

KEY POINTS

- Beef cattle veterinary practice focuses on providing service to the highly complex beef industry, producing food for consumers in a highly complex society.
- By incorporating thinking in systems, using the systems thinking discipline, beef cattle veterinarians can achieve better understanding, leading to increased relevance and impact.
- Systems thinking can be used to increase understanding of needs for the veterinary profession to advance.
- Attention to needs of students and new graduate beef cattle veterinarians to achieve practice readiness and successful onboarding are keys.
- Management of financial pressure, a substantial driver, might be addressed by focus on long-term solutions for sustainable progress.

INTRODUCTION

The range of veterinary medical services provided to the beef cattle industry has a history based somewhat on tradition, influenced by factors such as veterinarian–client relationships, success of services performed, and impact of services performed. The beef industry and veterinary medicine continue to evolve. There is increasing recognition of significant challenges to beef cattle veterinarians and their businesses.[1–4] Recruitment and retention of veterinarians in food animal practice and rural settings

[a] GPVEC- University of Nebraska-Lincoln, PO Box 148, Clay Center, NE 68933, USA; [b] GPVEC-University of Nebraska-Lincoln, PO Box 148, Clay Center, NE 68933, USA; [c] Livestock Veterinary Service, P.O. Box 353917 South Aurora Street, Eldon, MO 65026, USA; [d] College of Veterinary Medicine, University of Minnesota, 1365 Gortner Avenue Street, Paul, MN 55108, USA
* Corresponding author.
E-mail address: dgrotelueschen@unl.edu

Vet Clin Food Anim 38 (2022) 317–333
https://doi.org/10.1016/j.cvfa.2022.02.008
0749-0720/22/© 2022 Elsevier Inc. All rights reserved.

have become increasingly difficult.[5,6] Matching need to services provided often leaves gaps. Although individual animal focus plays a role in some livestock systems, transitioning to population-based approaches continues to be a change in progress in beef cattle veterinary practice.[6,7] Increased commitment to food systems is an increasingly important driver.[8] American Veterinary Medical Association (AVMA) membership data show 4861 and 4199 veterinarians listed in the food animal exclusive and food animal predominant sections of private clinical practice for 2012 and 2020, respectively, a 13.6% decrease, although there was an increase from 64,489 to 75,349 total veterinarians in private practice, a 16.8% change (**Fig. 1**).[9] Veterinarians listed in the private, clinical practice production medicine section of the AVMA census decreased to 3413 veterinarians in 2018 with reductions of 15.5% from 2008 to 2013 and 17.0% from 2013 to 2018.[10] Understanding of changes in the systems in which veterinary medicine and the beef industry participate, including food systems, is critical for appreciation of present realities and recognizing future opportunities for impact from services provided by veterinarians. Recognition of the beef industry as composed of highly and increasingly complex systems is essential to gaining understanding.

PERSPECTIVE ON THINKING IN SYSTEMS

The systems thinking discipline has significant potential to lead to better understanding, definition, and projection of roles of veterinarians and veterinary practices in the North American beef industry.[11] Traditional analytical approaches often break down complex subjects into pieces to enable better understanding of what is being considered. A cost of this approach is that perspective of the whole is lost. It can be rationalized that veterinary educations have historically and traditionally focused on these kinds of analytical approaches. Complexities of beef cattle veterinary practice, the beef industry and their roles in the food system require an in-depth understanding of the respective systems. Deeper understanding is imperative.[12]

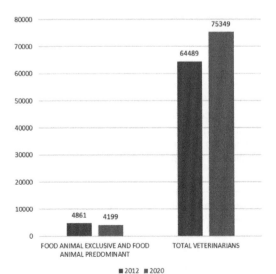

Fig. 1. Recent practice trends of AVMA Membership. (American Veterinary Medical Association. U.S. veterinarians 2020. https://www.avma.org/resources-tools/reports-statistics/market-research-statistics-us-veterinarians. Accessed September 15, 2021.)

It is essential that participants in systems associated with beef production understand the associated complexities. Systems thinking, as the systems thinking discipline, or simply, thinking in systems, can become a powerful resource for accomplishing this.[13] Engaging in systems or systems approaches does not necessarily mean engagement in formal systems thinking.

A system, defined by Meadows, is a set of elements or parts that is coherently organized and interconnected in a pattern or structure that produces a characteristic set of behaviors, often classified as its function or purpose.[14] Traditional education, including the field of veterinary medicine, has focused on linear thinking. An example is training that problem solving includes arrival at a specific diagnosis, with causation by a specific agent, such as a named bacterium, followed by the intervention that includes treatment and immediate or eventual resolution of the diagnosed condition. Most health issues experienced within beef cattle production systems are a result of risk factors superimposed on the system, resulting in immune-suppressed, susceptible animals that contract a resulting disease. This contrasts with linear thinking approaches. Most problems or crises are circular in nature, where actions or interventions implemented as solutions lead to unintended and often delayed consequences. The world is constructed into circular, interrelated systems with various levels of complexity. The methodologies of systems thinking significantly enhance our ability to gain awareness of how our actions often create feedback loops of unintended consequences. Because our interventions are often displaced in time and place from the negative results of the unintended consequences, our traditional linear approaches often fail to detect the interconnections of our actions.

Systems thinking has proven difficult to define at times. Jay Forrester is recognized as the father of the systems thinking discipline. He has stated that systems thinking has no clear definition or usage.[15] Forrester has stated that "systems thinking is coming to mean little more than thinking about systems, talking about systems, and acknowledging that systems are important. In other words, systems thinking implies a rather general and superficial awareness of systems."[15]

Other authors have attempted to attach definitions to systems thinking, with an example being a recently proposed definition published by Arnold. "Systems thinking is a set of synergistic analytic skills used to improve the capability of identifying and understanding systems, predicting their behaviors, and devising modifications to them to produce desired effects. These skills work together as a system."[16]

Consequences to systems thinking can lead to three outcomes. It provides an understanding of the existence and importance of systems, it leads to a deeper understanding of systems through systems dynamics, and negatively, can lead to misunderstanding if incomplete or lacking insights are used, and problem solving is not achieved or incorrect.[15] Because of the challenges surrounding complete and accurate understanding, systems thinking methodologies are often used iteratively over time to investigate observationally derived hypotheses. These "thought experiments" are effective tools of enlightenment and innovation; however, insights gained often may need further critical evaluation.

Rigor at the level of an academic discipline is needed to integrate systems thinking more fully into beef cattle veterinary medicine and the beef cattle industry. It is notable that multiple veterinary colleges have identified systems thinking education as a point of leverage in the training of future veterinarians. Systems thinking is an increasingly common topic addressed in production medicine rotations and graduate degree programs in many veterinary educational institutions. Scientific presentations and papers using systems thinking methodologies that were once rare are becoming more common.[17–20] It is also significant to note at least one professional veterinary program that the authors are aware of, teaches systems thinking and system dynamics in the first year, and reinforces it again during the clinical experience.[21] At the same time, terminology used in the systems thinking discipline can be difficult to specifically define. Terms can be quite conceptual and at times have not been routinely applied to scientific disciplines, especially veterinary medicine. Theories or hypotheses are traditionally applied in scientific settings. Systems include relationships and many other fields. Systems thinking terms can be interpreted differently and are adopted individually, due, in part to their conceptual nature and broad definition. Thus, systems thinking becomes a very expansive topic with potential for application by the user, whether an individual, a group, or another entity.

The primary goal of this article is to empower the reader to use a systems thinking process to understand challenges of beef cattle veterinary practice that might lead to the identification of leverage points leading to increased impact in the beef industry. This will be accomplished through the following approaches.

- To use systems thinking perspective to describe current realities of beef cattle veterinary practice in North America relative to its own complexities and in association with the beef cattle industry.
- To enable readers to gain a deeper understanding of beginning applications of systems thinking relative to beef cattle veterinary practice and the beef industry.

BEEF INDUSTRY SYSTEM BACKGROUND

Complexities in the beef industry are vast and increasing. Beef production and food systems have undergone immense change over time. Many aspects associated with supplying beef to consumers have changed dramatically as the food system has adapted. These range from beef animal production characteristics themselves to marketing of beef, segmentation, relationships with consumers, and consumption of beef. Relationships and involvements of the beef production industry continue to merge with food systems as needs and demands change. An example is the Beef Quality Assurance program, which communicates optimal production practices to consumers. Associated complexities continue to grow and change.

Consumer, environmental, and other issues are increasingly impacting production decisions. Beef cattle as ruminants are unique animals, with the ability to thrive by consuming large amounts of forage feedstuffs that are mostly unsuitable for other species, including humans. They are highly adaptable to diverse environments as they provide tremendous benefits to society.

Consequently, beef systems, ranging from animal production to aspects of the food system vary tremendously. Beef productions systems are extremely varied and individualized, influenced by characteristics such as goals of ownership, type of ownership, reasons for being in business, capitalization, size of the operation and business, rainfall and other environmental factors, proximity to markets, cost and availability of labor, and a host of other factors. Vertical and horizontal integration within production and food systems also increases complexity.

USDA National Agricultural Statistics Service (NASS) data for 2017 estimate 729,046 operations in the United Sates having beef cattle and calves. Data for 2007 estimate 764,984 farms and 1997 estimate 899,756 beef operations (**Fig. 2**).[22,23] These estimates represent a decrease of 19% over a 20-year period. For 2007, there were 607,708 farms with 1–49 beef cows, 84,253 farms with 50–99 beef cows, 67,210 farms with 100–499 beef cows, and 5813 farms with 500 or more beef cows, while in 2017 estimates report there were 576,735 farms with 1–49 beef cows, 80,411 farms with 50–99 beef cows, 65,962 farms with 100–499 beef cows, and 5938 farms with

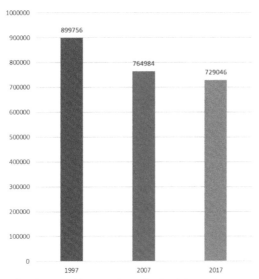

Fig. 2. Number of US beef cow-calf operations. (United States Department of Agriculture, National Agriculture Statistics Service, USDA/NASS Census of Agriculture historical highlights and earlier census years. Available at www.nass.usda.gov/Quick_stats/CDQT/Chapter/1/Table/1, accessed August 3 and 23, 2021)

500 or more beef cows (**Fig. 3**).[22,23] These data reflect decreases over the decade except for the category of herds with 500 or more beef cows, which showed a slight increase. These reflect national data. Local and statewide data should be examined as well.

Use of veterinary services seems to vary geographically in the United States. Use of veterinarians for specified consultative services over a 1-year period by cow/calf clientele was 51.9% for the western, 69.6% for the central, and 41.0% for eastern beef producers in the 2017 National Animal Health Monitoring Systems (NAHMS) Report.[24] Size of cow/calf operation influenced uses of specified veterinary consultative services as well with 47.2% of small operations (1–49 cows), 67.5% of medium operations (50–199 cows), and 76.9% of large operations (200 or more cows) using specified consultative services over a 1-year period in the 2017 NAHMS Report. The mean for all herds using these services over a 1-year period was only 52.8%.[24]

ADMIRING THE ICEBERG: IDENTIFYING CURRENT REALITIES, OBSERVATIONS, AND OPPORTUNITIES IN BEEF CATTLE VETERINARY PRACTICE

The beef industry has and continues to evolve significantly over time. Mental models, heavily influenced by tradition, have driven the structure of veterinary practices and services provided for decades. Ability and resolve of the veterinary profession to adapt, progress, and grow to positively impact food systems, including beef production and related systems, is an ongoing process. This article attempts to use systems thinking at elementary levels to begin discussion of application and problem solving relative to change in beef cattle veterinary practice. Much of the discussion reflects mental models related to traditional private, clinical veterinary practice engaged with beef cattle production. Future engagement with the beef industry by veterinarians could involve models not commonly found in today's settings. Recognition that

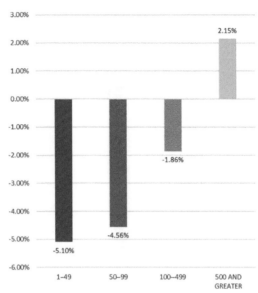

Fig. 3. Percent change in beef cow-calf operations based on herd size (2007–2017). (United States Department of Agriculture, National Agriculture Statistics Service, USDA/NASS Census of Agriculture historical highlights and earlier census years. Available at www.nass.usda.gov/Quick_stats/CDQT/Chapter/1/Table/1, accessed August 3 and 23, 2021.)

"practice" is legally defined in many states is acknowledged. Thinking in systems and with application to future beef cattle veterinary practice, a definition may be interpreted as "any graduate, licensed veterinarian engaged in some manner with the North American beef cattle industry," using a broad definition of "practice." Bias toward private clinical practice is acknowledged. However, other structures that meet the needs of the beef industry are also to be considered.

Seeking the understanding of the dynamics affecting change is important for future identification and implementation of leverage points to increase the impact of veterinary inputs into the beef industry. Examination of current realities of beef cattle veterinary practice is highly important. The iceberg framework provides a systems thinking approach to provide input into important questions.

- What are barriers to change in beef cattle veterinary practice?
- Why do we have the current realities?
- Why have these realities persisted?
- What are barriers to improvement?
- Why is relevance to the beef industry, despite large investments to prevent and address this, being asked?

Observations of the current realities of the iceberg help to identify shared perspectives and better identify root causes, which enable the identification of opportunities with leverage points for change. Events often drive thinking relative to addressing barriers. However, deeper introspection into patterns and systemic structures, that is, deeper into the iceberg, provides increased levels of understanding.

An exercise to gain more knowledge about the present realities of beef cattle veterinary practice was conducted by 17 members of the Veterinary Advancement of Systems Thinking (VAST) group by engaging in two sessions exploring the iceberg of present realities of beef cattle veterinary practice and observations and opportunities to achieve a desired state or vision. Characteristics of the group include 157 years (range 0–31 years) in private veterinary practice, 183.5 years (range 0–29 years) in academic setting, 49 years (range 0–21 years) in industry, and 2 years in federal service.

Current Realties of Beef Cattle Veterinary Practice

Participants were asked to briefly describe their highest concern about the present status of the veterinary profession relative to beef cattle practice followed by an oral discussion of expressed concerns. The following synopsis highlights points of discussion identified during the sessions that attempt to reflect the expressions of respective perceptions of participants.

Perspective: Structure of Practice Businesses/Practice Models

Structure of veterinary practice businesses or models has a tremendous impact on the success of each entity. Success may be interpreted in many ways, many of which are linked to financial outcomes and can include measures such as increasing gross income, increasing net income, growth to accommodate associates, and others. Success may also be measured by professional satisfaction, achievement of work–life balance, personal satisfaction factors, and others. Most measures of beef cattle veterinary practice success are impacted by the relevance of services provided. Examination of factors impacting success seems warranted.

- Financial stability is critical for the economic sustainability of beef veterinary practice businesses. Evaluation of options that present potential opportunities for practice growth to alleviate financial pressures is a part of practice management planning. These are variables depending on several factors. Some of these include veterinary expertise, passions, and interests of available veterinary expertise, geographic location, human populations, economic status of the area, financial viability of cow/calf, stocker, and feedlot enterprises and others. From a systems perspective, opportunities may result in the resolution of financial pressures by increasing revenue in the form of short-term fixes (**Fig. 4**). Implementation may include higher margin services and products. Examples might be increasing emphasis on other species and increasing product sales. However, these may severely limit the ability to evaluate client needs and improve match quality to enhance service and impact with present clientele. There are often time delays associated with long-term fixes, which might be more fulfilling financially and professionally. These require study and assessment of needs of the veterinary practice and the clientele businesses. Failure to address these aspects likely will decrease relevance and in the long-term will increase financial pressures.
- Apparent inability to advance existing practice structure to sustainable business models and retain practitioners in rural practices results in the lack of professional veterinary services available to our producers/production systems at levels that support their success long term (**Fig. 5**).
  - ○ Young practitioners leave to other practice types or focus due to dissatisfaction from inability to advance professional, personal, financial, and other goals.
  - ○ Existing practices are less able to attract or retain high-quality associates due to practice structure issues such as service models, hours worked, and financial sustainability.
  - ○ Production systems/producers are underutilizing veterinary services for high value/high return undertakings, thus undervaluing the veterinarian, and compounding ability to attract and retain new associates.

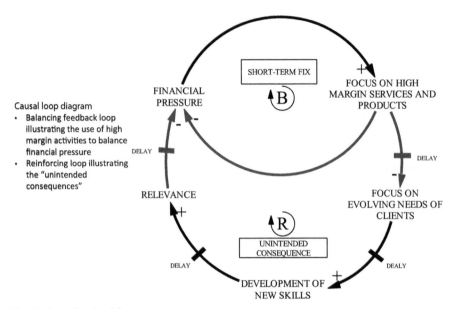

Fig. 4. Fixes that backfire.

Causal loop diagram
- Balancing feedback loop illustrating the use of high margin activities to balance financial pressure
- Reinforcing loop illustrating the "unintended consequences"

  o There is a lack of higher value services offered by practices and lack of client requests for these services that veterinarians can offer due to established "expectations" from previous veterinary experience.
- Financial remuneration is an important driver of structure for practice models. There is a serious question as to whether most fee structures are in alignment with sustainable practice models. Practice models that advance the financial interest of the practice based on treating sick animals are likely to be

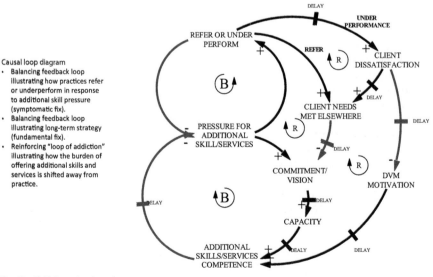

Causal loop diagram
- Balancing feedback loop illustrating how practices refer or underperform in response to additional skill pressure (symptomatic fix).
- Balancing feedback loop illustrating long-term strategy (fundamental fix).
- Reinforcing "loop of addiction" illustrating how the burden of offering additional skills and services is shifted away from practice.

Fig. 5. Shifting the burden.

fundamentally unsustainable. Traditional fee structures that are based on fixing or treating sick animals (a cost) rather than on the establishment of a process to prevent sick animals (value) lack alignment. A basic cost reduction approach by the producer, pressures for the removal of the veterinary cost in the production system, rather than seek return or value for investment in services.

- The structure of many practice models has reduced problem-solving capability with resulting compromises in services for beef cattle clientele. Root causes are likely related to economics and training along with the willingness to engage due to time commitment and ability. Using systems thinking to better understand, with approaches from a global perspective, gets to the fundamental root causes of problems our beef cattle clients have.

- Understanding of systems related to the beef industry and changes in veterinary practices addressing these are often neglected. There apparently are strong forces impacting practice models that result in a marginalized focus on client centricity. Financial pressures may be a causative factor. There are often long and protracted delays associated with rewards to efforts on client centricity and impacts on the practice, such as financial returns.

- Practice models generally have not developed to markedly promote the professional growth of veterinarians engaged in private beef cattle practice. This has impacted food animal veterinarians across the profession. The delay in the relevant skills and associated proficiencies taught in veterinary college and what will be relevant in the future has resulted in questions related to relevance. Other segments of veterinarians, such as swine and poultry, have developed practice structures that promote the development of new graduates and others into highly impactful, relevant veterinarians.

- The educational role of private practitioners is underused but highly important even though the information is widely available. Veterinarians are no longer the holders of information, and the profession has struggled at times with that reality. Practice models prioritizing education and delivery of information can reestablish veterinary practice businesses as primary resources.

- Priority on quality continuing education that contributes to personal mastery is critical. There is concern that the merit of many educational offerings may be compromised by intentional or unintentional biases of sponsors and presenters.

- Models often are not structured for new associates to introduce new services, which might increase the impact of the practice for clientele. Addition of new associates can address many aspects of generational change in a business. It is difficult for new associates to add new services in many traditional model practices.

Perspective: Impact and Relevancy to Beef Industry Clientele

There is concern that beef cattle veterinarians are becoming less relevant to beef producers and beef production systems. There is huge variability between beef enterprises that impacts the needs and wants of beef cattle clientele, including such aspects as herd size, geographic location, time in the beef business, goals of the enterprise, and other reasons. These should not be dismissed. The following observations were presented.

- The match quality of what our profession offers and what the beef system fundamentally needs is greatly lacking. Awareness by the veterinary profession in general seems to be lacking.

- Do we have an obligation to serve clients to who we perceive are engaged in unsustainable activities? It is necessary to decide who we want to be relevant to.
  - It is important to understand what type of client fits the sustainability model to your veterinary practice
  - The profession seems reluctant to change as an effort to keep pace with the system being served. Inclusion of clients in assessments of relevancy is highly important. Search for opportunities to better understand by also including different perspectives
- Are services being displaced by another provider, potentially at less cost? Clients expect traditional skills. However, other services can be more impactful.

Perspective: Veterinary Education and Training

There are strong mental models surrounding teaching and training that emphasize traditional skills. Training has focused strongly on individual animal treatment. Many veterinary colleges teach predominantly in a linear manner that instructs on traditional skills. Constraints in the educational system are recognizable and may benefit from in-depth systems analysis (**Fig. 6**).

Perspective: Attrition from Beef Cattle Veterinary Practice

Veterinarians are often more incentivized to move away from beef practice rather than expend the effort to adapt, or more concerningly, do not appreciate an avenue to adapt or change their current practice, and see exit from the practice as the only avenue to overcome the inertia of the current situation.

- Increased commitment to personal mastery, including scholarship is required. The development of new skill and/or knowledge in practice is an important aspect of practitioner growth and development within a practice. Although in many busy practices, it may be tempting to view continuing education as an expense or burden necessary to maintain licensure; it is instead an important avenue for developing and growing early-career practitioners.
- Agreement between skills emphasized during veterinary education and early practice can be a challenge for newly graduated practitioners. Newly graduated practitioners spend a great deal of time developing and becoming competent in additional technical skills and are judged by hiring practitioners and clients on their ability to service clients in a technical capacity. The ability to do this and develop trust with clients is an important aspect of early bovine practice; however, it can

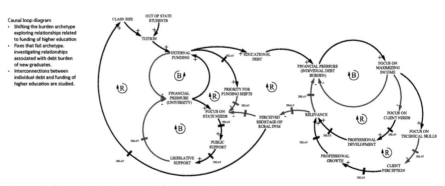

Fig. 6. Shifting the burden with fixes that fail.

present challenges for practitioners to transition out of the role of technical service provider and into a member of management teams as they mature in their practice career. A great deal of time is invested in veterinary school emphasizing the need for practitioners to leverage nontechnical skills in practice but do not always equip them with the tools to understand the process and transition that must occur to successfully implement those nontechnical aspects of practice.

- Attrition rate of young practitioners as they enter practice is related to multiple causes involving the individual and the practice. Practice models can be problematic, at times making it difficult for young veterinarians to evolve in their professional careers. Some practices lack approaches that provide value for clientele that can lead to eventual attrition by discouraged young practitioners.
- The economic structure of many practices, particularly cow-calf, is based on per head charge structure, making the addition of value-added services a challenge from a compensation perspective.
- Gaps in mentorship by experienced practitioners are often problematic.
- Quality of life expectations can be difficult to achieve. Included are cultural differences experienced by new graduates moving to new regions.

Perspective: New Graduates

Successful recruitment and onboarding of new graduates into beef cattle veterinary practice is undoubtedly one of the most important aspects of the future for practices. Graduation of candidates for these positions depends on several issues, one being admission into the veterinary college of students who possess a predictable likelihood of pursuing careers in beef cattle veterinary medicine.

- The priority of practices to successful onboarding of new veterinarians needs to be increased.
- Decreases are some service areas of practice due to changes in the beef industry can reduce young veterinarians' contact with beef cattle clientele. Examples include reduced brucellosis vaccination in the beef industry and reductions in the number of dystocias requiring Caesarean section surgeries. Threats to traditional pregnancy diagnosis services include blood-based tests for pregnancy and the availability of ultrasound capabilities.
- Inability to grow professional skills significantly 5–7 years after graduation becomes a deterrent to continuing in practice.
- Young graduates are subject to "sunk cost" bias early in their careers because they have so much invested; they feel like they must stick with the profession no matter what. They often settle for positions that provide a secure income rather than take professional and other risks.
- Young practitioners become comfortable offering basic technical tasks but lack the tools to transition offering high-value production medicine services.
  - Continuous improvement of curricula at veterinary colleges is needed to address these needs.
  - There is a lack of mentoring to help young practitioners develop this expertise early in their careers.

Perspective: Consumers and Societal Trends

Relationships between consumers and producers of food in agriculture can be improved. Beef cattle veterinarians can be a resource to play an intermediary role to educate and inform.

- Consumers as a group have less understanding of food production. This includes roles played by veterinarians. The societal role of beef cattle veterinarian continues to evolve.
- Observations were also made that consumers were more invested and engaged in providing input into food production methodologies and processes than in the past and a component of that input is to have veterinarians continue to play key roles.

Perspective: Trends in Agriculture and Food Production

Beef cattle veterinary medicine is in transition. Questions are raised about the profession's ability to adapt to changes in agriculture and food production in an impactful manner.

- Is our current relevance an indication that it is all the "system" currently requires? The US population has become much less agrarian, with less dependence on horses and mules for power inputs. Regulatory veterinary medicine played a larger earlier role but no longer does. How necessary are beef veterinarians?
- Industry consolidation will continue to define the role of veterinarians.
- Decreasing profit margins have pressured sustainability in agriculture and consequently veterinary medicine. Increasing levels of investment are required in production agriculture along with an exponential increase in complexity of production. Feedback from society into our "system" confirms changes are needed.
  - Despite the changes and the need to change, we still educate veterinarians in much the same ways as has been done in the past.
  - This has led to increased levels of highly educated specialists, often with less relevance to food production systems.
- Practice perspective
  - There are market indications that we are putting more veterinarians into practice than can thrive currently. Profit margins in beef production may be a limiting factor. An economic reality is that there may not be enough support for large supplies of rural veterinarians.
  - Does society prefer demands in the marketplace be left to determine supplies of veterinarians or should other fixes be applied to address perceived and real needs?

OBSERVATIONS AND OPPORTUNITIES FROM A SYSTEMS THINKING APPROACH

Participants were asked to engage in dialogue describing their desired state or vision for the beef cattle veterinary profession. These could include descriptions of future, highly relevant veterinary practices, the veterinary profession, veterinary education, obstacles to overcome, and other observations.

A present and future goal of beef cattle veterinarians is to achieve full alignment with the beef industry/beef producers to optimize capacity by accomplishing sustainability, productivity, efficiency, profitability, and resilience of the beef production system. In the language of systems thinking, this is known as the desired state. Required will be changes in mental models and priority emphasis on personal mastery.

Implementation of practice models that have strong client centricity is needed. This includes developing match quality to explore and address the needs of clientele and where needed, including providing leadership in communities and society.

- Practice models should be considered that have roles for professional expertise at tiered levels. These can be based on experience, levels of expertise, and certain areas of practice focus.

- Personal mastery is necessary so that veterinarians can be regarded as resources for information on technical skills, good husbandry practices, farm economics, marketing techniques, and nutrition questions. Veterinarians can be economically sustainable because of the information they provide.
- Change from the traditional mental model of reward for treating disease needs to change. Veterinarians should profit from health, not disease. Providing high-quality relevant information to clients to increase profitability is needed.
  - Veterinarians should aspire to compensation based on the maintenance of health and productivity together with sustainability of the environment and people resources without degradation of land and people. Search for models that achieve this.
- Veterinarians must search for ways to be adaptable to client needs, valued contributors to community, profession, and industry. Financial security is imperative such that debt does not limit options to provide value. Veterinarians should use their abilities to train others to be adaptable, resilient problem solvers.
- That individual animal health and population health and productivity is balanced within a system that is beneficial and matches the God-given resources of each unique organization.
- Veterinary medicine is hoped to continue to be a more personable profession, noted for the willingness to engage with people who are entrusted with the responsibility of raising livestock (beef cattle).

Emphasis on critical thinking skills in veterinary education is critical for students to learn about complex systems they will encounter in practice situations. Additionally, teaching to include personal mastery skills to better learn skills to better work with people, such as psychology, sociology, and communication, is needed.

Veterinary leadership and participation in components of the human food system are important. Private practitioners play key roles in the production of safe food. Trust in veterinarians as sources of information for consumers and clientele will enable credible communication between beef production and consumers. Increased participation by veterinarians at the interface between consumers and producers, providing an opportunity for improved communication, education, and other interactions.

A vision for veterinary medicine that results in more veterinarians who are passionate, engaged, and enthusiastic about our profession is a desired state. Facilitation of opportunity for private practitioners to evolve and grow in a scholarly way is a part of this state. Leaving a legacy of personal and professional satisfaction, honoring and upholding the veterinarian's oath, is an admirable goal accomplished by many veterinarians in previous and present generations. Maintaining generational values, quality of rural life and being good stewards of the things we are entrusted with insures successful achievement of this vision. To impart these values to clientele.

USING CAUSAL LOOP DIAGRAMS TO BETTER UNDERSTAND

Deeper understanding of the increasingly complex systems in which beef cattle veterinarians work is crucial for the profession to successfully adapt to change. Causal loop diagrams help to facilitate communication and understanding of relationships and forces that impact systems.[14] Previous chapters have addressed various aspects of the systems thinking discipline, which offers pathways to increase the ability to learn and communicate while thinking in systems. Although this article utilizes systems thinking in rather elementary forms, many additional tools are available.[13,14] It becomes evident that prioritization on practice models, which provide structure to the beef cattle veterinary practice, is fundamental. Study mental models[13] that address priorities such as match quality, personal mastery,[13] onboarding of new associates, practice readiness, client centricity, bias pitfalls introduced through financial structure and other forces, may be used to better adapt given achievement of deeper understanding.[13,14] Most of the perspectives provided by participants in the admiring the iceberg exercise are addressed in causal loop diagrams, which provide consideration to unintended consequences and other forces. Outcomes of the VAST group dialogue include the advancement of three causal loop diagrams that increase understanding of present realities in beef cattle veterinary practice (see **Figs. 4–6**).

The practice of veterinary medicine comes with many challenges and certainly meets the requirements to be considered a complex adaptive system, even when viewed from within its boundaries. In addition to the core professional responsibilities that define our profession such as conducting diagnostic investigations, managing disease outbreaks, designing, and implementing disease prevention plans, and managing the day-to-day operations of the practice, veterinarians owning and operating private practices also have the obligation to ensure the financial viability of the business venture itself. Financial pressure is a universal variable providing creative tension to the "system" that is a veterinary practice (see **Fig. 4**).

How the financial pressure is perceived and the time horizon for resolution of the creative tension is much influenced by experience, perspective, and magnitude and many other factors. Practice owners who could be considered "early" in their professional trajectory, for obvious reasons, are often subjected to the most intense financial pressure and consequently are under the most pressure to act decisively and quickly. Ability and aptitude in addressing financial pressure is an essential skill that supports the success of the practice and should not be overly criticized; however, the long-term implications of the tactics used in the short term to address financial pressure often goes unappreciated for many years.

From a systems thinking perspective, the long-term consequences can be more closely studied. In the short term, financial pressure is closely linked to profit margin derived from professional services and product sales, to balance the increase in financial pressure, a short-term fix would be to focus on services and products with the highest margin thereby relieving the financial pressure. However, when viewing the system from a longer time horizon, practitioners often reflect on the changes they have experienced over their career and see long-term financial sustainability more related to how well the services and products offered by the practice are valued by and fit the needs of the clients they serve. This match-quality alignment between what practice offers and what clients truly value and need to be successful can be seen as a powerful point of leverage. The delays associated with focusing on client needs and developing new skills to stay relevant are crucial to understanding. Because the relationship between the variables is often displaced by years to decades, it often goes unappreciated.

A central support model to highlight practice situations where there is a request for new or additional services that the practice has not offered or is unable to offer due to capacity or ability/skills is represented by a "Shifting the Burden" causal loop diagram (see **Fig. 5**). The immediate balancing loop action is to either refer to another entity that is able to provide or underperform or not provide the additional service, the long-term balance is to add the needed skillset or capacity, which is often associated with a delay. Following the referral option, the client will meet their needs elsewhere, creating a reinforcing loop and thus removing the pressure to offer the additional service by lowering the commitment or vision needed to add additional skillsets or capacity. Underperformance on the request in the short and long term can create reinforcing loops associated with client dissatisfaction that result in the client meeting needs elsewhere (similar to the referral loop) and issues with veterinary motivation that further contributes to decreasing the pressure to add capacity and ability/skills. This can result in the stagnation of practices and/or individual veterinarian's ability to evolve and veterinarian professional dissatisfaction that may lead to retention issues, all while continuing to not meet the requests/needs of clients.

A shortage of food supply veterinarians has occupied the attention of livestock producers, policy makers, and veterinary training institutions for more than a decade. Using a systems thinking approach, a causal loop diagram was generated to reflect a consensus of understanding reached by the VAST working group (see **Fig. 6**).

A focusing question was posed to the group. Why do food supply veterinary shortages remain persistent despite increases in veterinary training capacity designed to alleviate those shortages?

Two systems seem to interact to produce the perception of food supply veterinary shortages. On one side, new veterinarians encumbered with significant education debt seek employment and activities (especially in production-based compensation models) that are focused on maximizing income. Over time, these activities cause the new veterinarians to reduce focus on client needs and increase focus developing typical traditional skills to maintain income levels. The underlying mental model leading to these decisions often is, "I can't 'consult' straight out of veterinary school so I will focus on gaining expert proficiency in palpation, processing, and other highly technical skills." As client needs change, due to changing production environment, including social pressures, production scale, and other forces, there is a failure to invest in professional development activities that allow them to adapt along with their clientele. When client desire for veterinary participation in their production systems does not meet client expectations, the perception of a shortage of food supply veterinary capacity emerges.

In response to a decrease in the food supply veterinary capacity, veterinary schools have increased class sizes in attempts to satisfy public demands for food supply veterinarians. This response is an apparent win–win because financial pressure in university systems is routine and is often addressed by increasing revenue from sources other than traditional state appropriations, which would be typical for land-grant universities. Tuition is an important source of external revenue for veterinary schools facing financial pressures, such budget cuts, and the ability to increase class sizes for the good of society while mitigating economical strain is appealing. One notable problem that has emerged is the frequency and magnitude of substantial indebtedness associated with a veterinary education. The change in indebtedness is multifactorial but is partially explained by the frequency of students attending out-of-state schools and the rising cost of veterinary education. The educational debt increases the pressure on veterinarians to maximize income early in efforts to reduce debt and position themselves for other costly endeavors like purchasing a practice and/or a home.

Veterinary schools have leveraged the shortage of food supply veterinarians to increase training capacity and develop alternative training methods to increase the supply of food animal veterinarians in underserved areas. As previously stated, this solution provides veterinary schools to demonstrate an effort in response to a prominent public concern.

Our hypothesized answer to the focusing question is that as veterinarians lose relevance to their clients through a focus on veterinary services that maximize income to the veterinary rather than on services that help clients succeed in a changing environment, livestock producers perceive a lack of veterinary support for their operations that has been labeled a "shortage of food supply veterinarians." Pressure on elected officials and veterinary schools has resulted in expansions of training capacity designed to produce a sufficient number of veterinarians to satisfy producers' desire for veterinary support. Unfortunately, much, or most of the expansion has been achieved through the enrollment of nonresident students. This fact coupled with the increasing cost of veterinary education has resulted in an increase in the frequency and indebtedness of graduate veterinarians, which drives behavior aimed at maximizing income. If our hypothesis is correct, any behavior that increases veterinary student indebtedness is likely to produce an accelerating perception of food supply veterinary service shortage. Likewise, focus on alleviation of this shortage by increasing the supply of veterinarians will actually amplify the problem.

SUMMARY

Increased understanding of the complexities of beef cattle veterinary medicine by becoming competent in systems thinking, including the systems thinking discipline, can be an important and powerful tool for developing beef veterinary practice having high match quality that delivers impactful services to the beef industry. Personal mastery includes a wide array of knowledge and skills and involves understanding of food systems, in which the beef industry participates. Incorporation of systems thinking into veterinary training curricula offers good potential for improving new graduate preparedness for practice. Increased focus on practice readiness,[25] including mentorship at multiple levels,[26] and onboarding of new and recent graduates would help to address match quality and attrition issues. Many current models used in beef cattle veterinary practice interfere and conflict with sustainability and achievement of professional and personal goals. Many of the fundamental concerns about the relationships of beef cattle veterinary medicine with the beef industry can be improved by focus on match quality, addressing mismatches between services offered and the services needed for long-term sustainability of veterinary practices.

DISCLOSURE

Three authors (D.M. Grotelueschen, J.T. Groves, and B. Vander Ley) have received honoraria to provide education on the topic of Systems Thinking to veterinarians. The other authors have nothing to disclose.

ACKNOWLEDGMENTS

The authors wish to thank the 17 members of the VAST group who contributed their valuable perspectives through the "admiring the iceberg" exercises and advancement of causal loop diagrams in this article.

REFERENCES

1. Hoblet KH, Maccabe AT, Heider LH. Veterinarians in population health and public practice: Meeting critical national needs. J Vet Med Ed 2002;30:232–9.
2. Osborn BI, Kelly AM, Salman MD, et al. Crisis in veterinary medicine. JAVMA 2021;258:704–6.
3. National Research Council. Workforce needs in veterinary medicine. Washington (DC): The National Academies Press; 2013. p. 57–90.
4. Ruston A, Shortall O, Green M, et al. Challenges facing the farm animal veterinary profession in England: a qualitative study of veterinarians' perceptions and responses. Prev Vet Med 2016;127:84–93.
5. Cast Issue 67 Task Force Members. Impact of recruitment and retention of food animal veterinarians on the U.S. food supply. CAST Issue Paper 2020;67:1–16.

6. Barrington GM, Allen AJ. Food animal veterinarians: Where we came from and where we might go. Online J Rural Res Policy 2010;5:1–7.
7. Larson RL. Food animal veterinary medicine: Leading a changing profession. J Vet Med Ed 2004;31:341–6.
8. Hurd HS. Food systems veterinary medicine. Anim Health Res Rev 2011;12: 187–95.
9. American Veterinary Medical Association. U.S. veterinarians. 2020. Available at: https://www.avma.org/resources-tools/reports-statistics/market-research-statistics-us-veterinarians. Accessed September 15, 2021.
10. Ouedrago FB, Bain B, Hansen C, et al. A census of veterinarians in the United States. JAVMA 2019;255:183–91.
11. Duboz R, Echaubard P, Panomsak P, et al. Systems thinking in practice: Participatory modeling as a foundation for integrated approaches to health. Front Vet Sci 2018;5:1–8.
12. Sinek S. Start with why. New York: Penguin Group; 2009. p. 11–34.
13. Senge PM. The fifth discipline. New York: Crown Business; 2006. p. 6–12.
14. Meadows DH. Thinking in systems. White River Junction (VT): Chelsea Green Publishing; 2008. p. 188.
15. Forrester J. Systems dynamics, systems thinking, and soft OR. Syst Dyn Rev 1994;10:245–56.
16. Arnold RD. Definition of systems thinking: a systems approach. Proc Comp Sci 2015;44:669–78.
17. Groves JT. Details to attend to when managing high-risk cattle. Vet Clin Food Anim 2020;35:445–60.
18. Larson RL. Systems thinking and beef cattle production medicine: issues of health and production efficiency. Food Safety, Elsevier; 2015. p. 421–6.
19. Smith DR. Risk factors for bovine respiratory disease in beef cattle. Anim Health Res Rev 2020;21:149–52.
20. Rethorst D. Flippin' the iceberg: A systems thinking approach to immunology and vaccination protocols in beef cow-calf systems. AABP Recent Graduate Conf Proc 2021;54:90–7.
21. Smith DR. Mississippi State University, Personal Communication, September 23, 2021.
22. United States Department of Agriculture, National Agriculture Statistics Service, USDA/NASS Census of Agriculture historical highlights and earlier census years. Available at: www.nass.usda.gov/Quick_stats/CDQT/Chapter/1/Table/1. Accessed August 3 and 23, 2021.
23. United States Department of Agriculture, National Agriculture Statistics Service. Livestock operations, final estimates 2003-2007, Statistical bulletin 1021, 2009.
24. United States Department of Agriculture. Beef 2017: beef cow/calf management practices in the United States 2017, report 1. USDA-APHIS-VS-CEAH-NAHMS. Fort Collins (CO).#.782.0520. 2020. pp 87-89.
25. Fingland RB, Stone LR, Read EK, et al. Preparing veterinary students for excellence in general practice: building confidence and competence by focusing on spectrum of care. JAVMA 2021;259:463–70.
26. Furr MO, Raczkoski BM. Perceptions of training, self-efficacy, and mentoring among veterinary clinical specialty trainees. JAVMA 2021;259:528–38.

Printed and bound by CPI Group (UK) Ltd, Croydon, CR0 4YY

03/10/2024

01040470-0015